# *Handbook to Live Well with Adhesive Arachnoiditis*

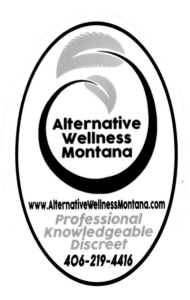

Published by *"Arachnoiditis Research and Education Project"*
*Tennant Foundation.* Copyright© 2019 Forest Tennant MD, MPH, DrPH

First Printing: 2019
ISBN: 9781700411709

Arachnoiditis Research and Education Project
c/o Nancy Kriskovich
14 Hidden River Lane
Bigfork, MT 59911

Ordering Information:

Special discounts are available on quantity purchases by corporations, associations, educators, and others. For details, contact the publisher at the above listed address.

U.S. trade bookstores and wholesalers: Please contact Nancy Kriskovich Tel: (406)249-2002;
or email snkriskovich@gmail.com

All proceeds from the sale of this book will go to the Arachnoiditis Research and Education Project sponsored by the
TENNANT FOUNDATION.
336 ½ S. GLENDORA AVENUE
WEST COVINA, CA 91790-3060
A 501(c)(3) Non-profit Organization

# About the Authors

### Dr. Forest Tennant Biography 2019

Dr. Forest Tennant has had a long, distinguished career in addiction and pain medicine. He was recently honored with a "Life-Time Achievement Award" by Pain Week and "50 Years of Service" by the journal, "Practical Pain Management" where he served as their medical editor for 12 years. Dr. Tennant began his career in addiction and pain medicine as a US Army medical officer during the Vietnam War Era at which time he helped develop the Army's drug testing, education and treatment programs. After the Vietnam War, he became a Public Health Fellow assigned to the UCLA School of Public Health where he obtained his Masters' and Doctorate in Public Health (MPH, DrPH). Since 1975 to the present day, Dr. Tennant has produced a steady flow of research and publications in addiction and pain medicine. During this time his public notoriety first emerged when he served as an expert witness in the criminal trials of the physicians of Howard Hughes and Elvis Presley. Later he developed the drugs of abuse and anabolic steroid testing programs for the Los Angeles Dodgers and the National Football League. In very recent years Dr. Tennant has chosen to research hormonal testing and treatment of intractable pain and the merging pain problems of adhesive arachnoiditis and genetic collagen disorders. He and his wife Miriam of 52 years reside and work in West Covina, California and Wichita, Kansas.

### Ingrid Hollis Biography 2019

Ingrid Hollis began her career as a classically trained artist. This life path was put on hold by the necessity of becoming a family caregiver. This experience, along with a life altering motor vehicle accident in 1996 and the discovery that she has hypermobile Ehlers Danlos syndrome, (hEDS), a genetic collagen disorder that also runs in her family, changed the direction of her life. This knowledge set her on a course to search for answers, medical help and cures.

A great curiosity for research was ignited through this direct experience and fueled the desire to help others in similar situations. She has studied traditional and non-traditional medicine from many remarkable physicians and healers from throughout the world. Her hope has been to glean the wisdom from the many different healing systems and find ways to help and improve the lives of persons and their families who suffer from rare diseases throughout the world.

Ingrid resides in Colorado with her retired husband and son. She has two lovely children and two grandchildren to whom her work is dedicated.

She heads the "Publication Team" for the Arachnoiditis Research and Education Project of the Tennant Foundation.

# CONTRIBUTORS

A handbook as comprehensive as this could not have been written without the input and advice of many people. We are grateful for the kind assistance of those persons listed here.

Terri Anderson
Lynn Ashcraft
Donna Corley
Lloyd Costello, MD
K. Scott Guess, PharmD, MS Pharm, RPh
Adam Hy, DO
Kate Lamport
Denise Molohon
Kristen Ogden
Caron Pedersen RN, NP, DC
Martin J. Porcelli, DO, MHPE
Rhonda Posey
Gary Snook
Deborah Vallier
Kris Walters

This handbook and the research behind it would never have been written without the pioneering groundwork of Drs. Sarah Smith, Antonio Aldrete, and Charles Burton.

# *Handbook to Live Well with Adhesive Arachnoiditis*

## BY

## FOREST TENNANT M.D., M.P.H., DR.P.H
## with INGRID HOLLIS

# Table of Contents

## INTRODUCTION AND PURPOSE

This handbook has one purpose – to help you live well despite this horrible disease: adhesive arachnoiditis (AA).

We first encountered AA in the 1970's when insoluble dyes (usually "pantopaque") was injected into the spinal canal to help visualize x-rays. Today the causes are different, and AA is increasing in the general population.

AA is a complex neuroinflammatory disease of the spinal canal covering (arachnoid) and the lumbar spinal cord nerve roots (cauda equina). In other words, two different body parts abnormally "glue" together by adhesions. Regardless of cause, AA, once initiated, can be a, progressive disease that can result in constant severe pain, paralysis of arms and legs, and impairments of bladder, bowel, and sex organs. Due to the increasing prevalence of AA, the Tennant Foundation has initiated a vigorous and aggressive research project to understand and develop strategies and protocols to control and treat AA. While no absolute cure is known, we have determined that AA is best treated and controlled with a two-fold strategy: (1) medication and (2) physiologic and preventive measures.

We have recently learned that persons with genetic collagen disorders of the Ehlers-Danlos Syndrome and Marfan Syndrome types frequently develop AA. This handbook addresses our efforts to bring treatment to those with this dual disease problem.

Today, few physicians are aware and familiar with the strategies to control AA which is a major reason this handbook has been written. Although we predict a change in the future, we have learned that people with AA and their families must currently initiate treatment pretty much on their own. To wait can be a terrible mistake, since AA can swiftly progress and worsen causing deterioration and lead to a miserable, shortened life. This handbook is primarily designed to keep people with AA from getting worse, but there is hope as most people get better with the measures outlined in this handbook. Plunge in. Even when you find good medical care for AA, you will have to practice measures described in this handbook.

Forest Tennant M.D., Dr. P.H.
Ingrid Hollis

## WHY WERE OUR CAST OF CHARACTERS CREATED?

Adhesive arachnoiditis (AA) is an extremely serious disease and not to be taken lightly; however, we have created some characters to emphasize certain points of importance. It is our intent to bring a smile along with getting important points across to the reader.

### DR. BEAK

Who is Dr. Beak? A smart old buzzard who received his MD degree from the "Common Sense Medical School." He will give common sense advice.

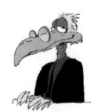

### NURSE ROSEY

Who is Nurse Rosey? A pesky, ever present nurse who wrote her nurse's thesis on "How to Shape Up Persons for Their Own Good." She will give you gentle, compassionate, encouragement.

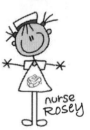

### HAPPY SPIDER

How can a spider be happy? Well, it is his web of arachnoid tissue that becomes inflamed with AA. Spiders are meticulous about their web and when you allow his web to be distorted with inflammation, he becomes unhappy. He can be happy when you are following the protocol and his web is no longer inflamed and causing you pain.

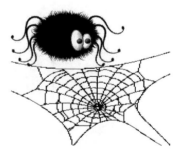

[14]

# 1. MAJOR MESSAGE – BUILD A PERSONAL CARE PROGRAM

Every person who has adhesive arachnoiditis (AA) and obtains this handbook is undoubtedly aware that this disease can result in tragedy, pain, and suffering beyond imagination. A meaningful life can stop on a dime if AA develops and it is not controlled.

Our major message is this. You can build a personal care program that controls this disease and lets you live a quality, meaningful life. It's not, however, easy. You must build a program of medication and physiologic measures. You can't do it all in one day or in a couple of visits to a doctor's office, but it will happen with a little effort and discipline. You must build a program step by step and self-administer and practice your program daily with a goal of improvement, while constantly enhancing your program.

Here are cautions to know while building your program. Relief of pain is usually the paramount concern of a person with AA. This is understandable but, know this: any medication called a pain reliever – prescription or non-prescription – will only provide relief for a limited time period unless you are simultaneously taking medication to suppress neuroinflammation and medication agents to regrow damaged nerve tissue. You must also practice some of the physiologic and preventive measures in this handbook if you want consistent pain relief.

A second caution is this. Modern medicine has done a masterful job in selling a single treatment for a single disease. Media, print, TV, and the internet are constantly trying to sell the "new" stuff like stem cells, microsurgery, minimally invasive spine surgery, robotic surgery, intravenous infusions, and hyperbaric oxygen chamber treatment among others. While all these may have merit in select clinical situations, there is no substitute for an effective AA care plan which requires medications and specific physiologic measures designed to reduce neuroinflammation, regrow your damaged nerve tissue, and keep you mobile, animated, and living a quality life.

The last caution is to avoid some buzz words used to describe treatments that are usually designed for someone's financial gain or disguised as cost saving measures by insurance carriers and HMO's. Look out for "evidence-based", "person-centered", and "off-label" cures. Check all the "one-way" or "no-way" words. Don't let propaganda keep you from building an effective treatment program.

## 2. DEALING WITH THE FRIGHT OF AA

Every person who is informed they have AA is rightfully scared and frightened. To be otherwise would not be human. When one has severe pain, spasms, funny feelings on the skin, an irregular bladder, and blurred vision you will naturally be scared.

What's more, the stories of the past – paralysis, starvation, horrific pain, non-functioning mind and body, and early death were all true at one time, but no more! Our medical protocols for AA aren't totally curative, but because of them the plight of AA victims in the past doesn't have to occur today.

Follow these steps:

1. Don't let fright paralyze you or cause you not to act. You must take immediate action once you find out you've got AA.

[16]

2. Tell someone about your fright – spouse, friend, child, doctor, clergyman – nothing calms fright like sharing it with another person.

3. Understand this new medical fact – modern treatment as outlined in this handbook will almost always keep you from getting much worse – just start. Bottom line – get started with treatment today!

4. First treatment – take a walk – walking is a first-class medicine for AA. Second, go to the health food store and buy one or two non-prescription drugs known to help most people with AA– examples: curcumin, serrapeptase, pregnenolone.

5. Make an appointment with your family doctor, nurse practitioner (NP), or physician assistant (PA) to discuss treatment strategies.

6. Take out a pencil and paper. Write down every medication, food, exercise, or posture that gives you some comfort. You will be surprised. You already know some things that will help you live a good life!

The best way to rid yourself of fright is to know your challenges and that you have the power to control AA!

# 3. DEFINITIONS YOU MUST KNOW

Adhesive Arachnoiditis (AA): This condition is present when there are adhesions between the arachnoid layer and the nerve roots in the cauda equina. Adhesions "glue" the nerve roots to the arachnoiditis layer, and this can be seen on a magnetic resonance image (MRI).

Fundamentally AA is the abnormal "gluing" together of two different body parts, the lumbar nerve roots and spinal canal covering.

Arachnoid: The cover or lining of the spinal canal is scientifically called the thecal sac or meninges. The inner layer is called the "Pia Mater". It is extremely thin and fragile. The outer layer is the dura which is thick and firm. The arachnoid is the middle layer. It contains blood vessels and inflammatory cells and can become inflamed if irritated or damaged.

Central Nervous System (CNS): CNS is the brain, spinal cord, and cauda equina nerve roots.

Cerebral Spinal Fluid (CSF): Fluid made in the brain that bathes, protects, and nourishes the spinal cord and brain.

Medication Dosage: Milligram is mg. Milliliter is ml.

Nerve Roots: The actual spinal cord runs from the brain down to the top of the lumbar area. Below the spinal cord hangs about 2 dozen string-like structures called nerve roots. Collectively they are called the cauda equina. The nerve roots can become damaged, inflamed, clump together, and stick or adhere by adhesions to the arachnoid layer of the spinal canal cover. When sticking and adhesions occur, the term AA is applied. If only enlargement, displacement, and clumping of nerve roots is seen on MRI, the term "cauda equina syndrome" is sometimes applied. Symptoms can be similar to AA.

Neuroinflammation (NI): NI is inflammation that occurs inside the CNS. It is the basic cause of AA and must be suppressed if an AA person is to control AA.

Neuroregeneration or Neurogenesis (NR): NR is regrowth of damaged nerve tissue, including nerve roots and supporting cells called glia.

Spinal Canal: The spinal canal is fundamentally a pipe that contains 4 components: (1) spinal cord; (2) nerve roots; (3) covering or lining called the meninges; and (4) cerebral spinal fluid. Think of the spinal canal as a closed pipe filled with structures bathed in fluid.

Tarlov Cysts: A cyst or outpouching of a spinal nerve root. They are often called "perineural" cysts. Tarlov cysts are frequently associated with ARC/AA.

Three Component Medical Treatment of AA: (1) suppression of neuroinflammation, (2) promotion of neuroregeneration, and (3) pain control.

Troche: Medication in a dissolvable Tablet or Lozenge that goes between the tongue and cheek.

Two Strategies for Treatment of AA: (1) medication and (2) physiologic measures.

# 4. HISTORY OF ARACHNOIDITIS

AA is an old disease first recognized in the mid-1800's (19th Century). The causes in that century were primarily the infections of tuberculosis and syphilis. Fortunately, these diseases almost disappeared in the 20th century because antibiotics were discovered that dramatically reduced their prevalence. In the 20th century the major cause of AA was insoluble dyes injected into the spinal canal to enhance x-rays for diagnostic purposes. In 1987, the MRI was invented which lead to the near extinction of AA. In modern times (the 21$^{st}$ century) AA, has re-emerged due to numerous factors including aging, degenerative spine conditions, obesity, and excessive sitting before computers and television screens, and invasive spine interventions and surgeries, among other factors.

- The word "arachnoid" refers to a spider's web because the arachnoid membrane resembles one.

- The exact year the disease, "arachnoiditis," was named is uncertain, however, the 1873 "Comprehensive Medical Dictionary," published by J.B. Lippincott & Co., included this definition of arachnoiditis: "A faulty term, denoting inflammation of the arachnoid membrane."

- In 1869 the famous neurologist, Dr. Charcot and his colleagues first described a syndrome we now call the disease, ARC. The causes of the disease were infections, primarily tuberculosis and syphilis.

- Dr. Addison, the physician who discovered adrenal failure, published his findings on 11 autopsied cases in 1855. Two cases had severe pain, atrophied adrenals with calcium deposits, and fluid around the arachnoid layer, which suggested that long-standing, end-stage ARC was a likely cause of pain and adrenal failure.

- The first recorded attempt to treat AA was probably in 1781 when Dr. John Fothergill, a renowned British physician, treated a person with severe back and sciatic pain who had other symptoms compatible with AA.  Opioids had failed to relieve this person's pain, but he obtained positive results with a mercury concoction called calomel.

- Between about 1930 and 1990 pantopaque and other oil-insoluble dyes were infused into the spinal canal for diagnostic (myelogram) purposes.  A small percentage of these people developed AA and other neurologic complications.

- MRI's replaced oil-based dyes in the late 1980's, and AA subsequently became a rare, unappreciated disease.

- Beginning around the year 2000, an extended life span, with increasing rates of chronic painful spinal conditions such as herniated discs and arthritis. This along with the increasing use of invasive medical interventions and surgeries to treat them, began fueling a rise in the incidence and prevalence of AA that continues to this day.

# 5. AA IS INCREASING IN MODERN TIMES

- Until recently AA was considered an extremely rare disease.  NO MORE.  Thanks to the technology of MRI's, AA can be diagnosed in a person with typical history, symptoms, and physical exam.

- While most cases of AA are in the lumbar and sacral spine areas, it can also occur in the cervical (neck) and thoracic (chest) spine. Although there are only a few nerve roots in the cervical and thoracic spine, the arachnoid layer of the spinal canal covering in these spinal areas can become chronically inflamed and produce profound pain and disability. Rarely do adhesions form between the spinal cord and arachnoid lining in the cervical and thoracic areas.

- It now appears that many people who have been labeled with such subjective, non-specific terms like "degenerative spine," "low back pain" or "failed back syndrome" really have AA.

Factors Leading to AA:

- ✓ Sedentary (sitting) lifestyle*
- ✓ Poor posture
- ✓ Non-supportive footwear
- ✓ Bucket seats
- ✓ Risk-taking sports activities
- ✓ Obesity
- ✓ Lack of exercise and walking
- ✓ Risky spinal injections and surgery
- ✓ Longer lifespan and aging
- ✓ Emergency life saving measures following accidents**
- ✓ Increased infant and childhood survival rates due to antibiotics and vaccines***

*Refers to the long hours of sitting in front of television and computers
**Life may be saved but injury left behind
***Immune deficient infants may survive and develop tissue degeneration disorders in adulthood

| The normal anatomy of the spinal cord and nerve roots |
| --- |

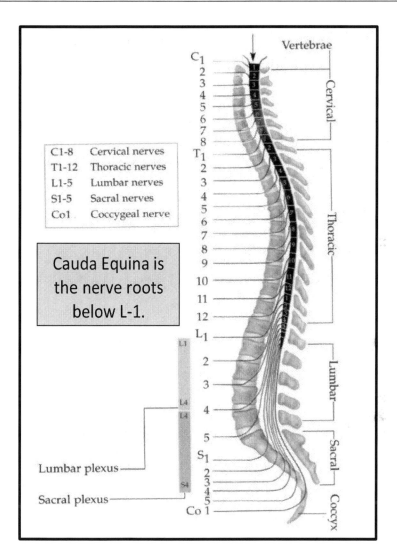

| C1-8 | Cervical nerves |
| --- | --- |
| T1-12 | Thoracic nerves |
| L1-5 | Lumbar nerves |
| S1-5 | Sacral nerves |
| Co1 | Coccygeal nerve |

Cauda Equina is the nerve roots below L-1.

Lumbar plexus

Sacral plexus

Vertebrae
Cervical
Thoracic
Lumbar
Sacral
Coccyx

# 6. CAUSES OF ADHESIVE ARACHNOIDITIS

✓ In the 1800's the common causes of AA were the infections of tuberculosis and syphilis.

[23]

✓ In the 1900's the most common cause of AA was oil-based dyes injected into the spinal canal for diagnostic purposes.

✓ In the 2000's the most common causes are chronic spine disorders related to aging, accidents, obesity, bucket seats, lack of exercise, poor posture, and the invasive medical interventions and procedures that are now used to treat common spine disorders.

Listed Here are the Common Causes of AA Today:

Common Spine Disorders

Common spine disorders including chronic herniated discs, stenosis, osteoporosis, and vertebral arthritis may, over-time, cause nerve roots in the cauda equina to rub or be squeezed together causing friction "sand-paper effect," inflammation, and adhesions.

Genetic Collagen Disorders

The arachnoid and pia mater layers of the spinal covering are thin, soft, and easily damaged because they are composed primarily of very soft and frail tissue compared to other tissues such as tendons and bone. Genetic collagen disorders that cause tissue degeneration, particularly Ehlers-Danlos and Marfan Syndromes, may cause micro-tears in the arachnoid layer which lead to inflammation, cysts (Tarlov), and adhesions.

Autoimmune Disease

Many people with AA also have autoimmune diseases such as systemic lupus, psoriatic arthritis, or rheumatoid arthritis. AA may be a direct result from autoimmunity.

Infections

Lyme disease is the most common infection today that may cause AA. Some viruses are also highly suspected to cause AA. Epstein Barr virus is one possibility.

Trauma

A puncture, tear, or traumatic injury to the arachnoid lining from an accident, needle puncture, or chemical irritant may initiate AA. Inflammation and adhesions of the arachnoid lining may later capture, glue and inflame the nerve roots that are close to the traumatic site.

# 7. NATURAL COURSE AND OUTCOME OF ADHESIVE ARACHNOIDITIS

3 Possible Outcomes of Untreated AA:

- Resolves – a return to the normal uninflamed state (mild or asymptomatic cases)
- Intermittent symptoms, impairments, and pain
- Progressive neurologic symptoms, impairments, and pain (e.g. wheelchair, bed-bound, early death)

AA's natural course and outcome are directly related to neuroinflammation severity. Due to this fact, suppression of neuroinflammation along with neuroregenerative measures is the "baseline" of treatment.

## 8. WHY PREMATURE DEATH OCCURS IN PEOPLE WITH AA

- Poor mobility
- Obesity, diabetes, hypercholesterolemia
- Endocrine (hormone) suppression
- Immune system impairment - inability to protect against disease from infections and tumors
- Hypertension
- Intestinal digestive defects, gastroparesis, and malabsorption – inability to absorb needed nutrients from food

The Good News:  We now know that the natural course and outcome of AA CAN BE greatly changed by treating neuroinflammation and promoting neuroregeneration.

## 9. MAJOR SYMPTOMS AND HARMS OF AA

Due to nerve entrapment and destruction of nerve roots, these major symptoms may appear: (1) skin sensation of water dripping or bugs crawling, (2) burning feet, (3) can't sit or stand in one position very long, (4) bladder difficulties, and (5) pain.

[26]

Additional symptoms may occur due to AA's complications:

- ✓ Spinal Fluid Flow Obstruction: headache, blurred vision, ringing in ears
- ✓ Spinal Fluid Leakage: back pain, decreased ability to extend arms and legs, difficulty walking
- ✓ Autoimmune Disorder: arthritis, muscle aches, cardiac disorders, seizure, thyroiditis, carpal tunnel
- ✓ Retained Electricity: vibrations, tremors, overheating episodes, sweating, jerking
- ✓ Hormone Suppression; weakness, fatigue, poor pain control, depression, tissue wasting

Key Message: The sooner treatment with anti-neuroinflammation agents is started reduction in symptoms and harm can start.

# 10. CATEGORIES OF SEVERITY

AA has different severities, and we divide the severity into 4 categories: (1) mild; (2) moderate; (3) severe; and (4) catastrophic. Below we list the categories with impairments and functions in each category. If you are in the mild or moderate category, you have an excellent chance of considerable recovery. In fact, you may not even require a prescription drug if you are in the mild category. If you are in the severe or catastrophic categories, you will need a full protocol with the most potent drugs, and you may even need an implanted electrical stimulator or intraspinal opioid pump to get adequate pain relief.

Mild:
- ✓ Full range of motion
- ✓ No back indentation or contracture

- ✓ Normal inflammatory markers
- ✓ No bladder impairment
- ✓ No MRI evidence of spinal fluid leakage or obstruction
- ✓ No hormone abnormalities
- ✓ Can sit and stand in one position for 10 minutes

Moderate:
- ✓ Full range of motion and walks without assistance
- ✓ Mild to zero lower extremity weakness
- ✓ Normal inflammatory markers
- ✓ Some bladder hesitancy, urgency, dripping
- ✓ No MRI or physical evidence of spinal fluid leakage
- ✓ Mild constant pain but no need for sleep medication
- ✓ Can sit and stand in one position for 10 minutes

Severe:
- ✓ Some range of motion impairment and needs assistance (cane or other) to ambulate
- ✓ Weakness in lower extremities with neurologic symptoms (e.g. burning feet, bugs crawling, jerking or other)
- ✓ Elevated inflammatory markers and/or hormone abnormalities
- ✓ Bladder impairment symptoms of hesitancy, urgency, or incontinence
- ✓ MRI and/or physical evidence of chronic spinal fluid leakage and/or flow obstruction
- ✓ Constant pain that impairs sleep
- ✓ Can't sit and stand in one position for 10 minutes

Catastrophic:

- ✓ Requires assistance with activities of daily living (dressing, toiletry, eating, etc.)
- ✓ Significant lower extremity impairment (needs walker, wheelchair, braces)
- ✓ Bladder impairment of hesitancy, urgency, or incontinence
- ✓ Mental deficiencies such as memory loss or reading ability
- ✓ MRI and physical evidence of chronic spinal fluid obstruction and leakage
- ✓ Elevated inflammatory markers and hormone abnormalities
- ✓ Constant pain that impairs sleep
- ✓ Can't sit or stand in one position for 10 minutes

# 11. DIAGNOSIS OF AA

A final, clinical diagnosis of AA requires typical symptoms, physical findings, and laboratory tests.  An MRI is needed to confirm the diagnosis.

Here is a 7-question screen.  We have found that if a person answers yes to 4 of the 7, they very likely have AA.  The earlier the diagnosis in the course of the disease, the better the results of treatment.

1. In addition to chronic pain, do you ever experience sharp, stabbing pains in your lower back when you twist, turn or bend?
2. Do you ever experience bizarre skin sensations such as crawling insects or water dripping down **one or both legs**?
3. Do you ever have burning, tingling, or a sensation of walking on broken glass in your feet and/or toes?
4. Does your pain become worse after standing, sitting, and/or walking?

5. Do you have leg weakness and/or pain that radiates down one or both legs?
6. Do you experience any bladder dysfunction such as dribbling, or difficulty when starting or stopping urination?
7. Do you have headaches along with blurred vision?

If you answered yes to four or more of these seven questions, you most likely have AA or some other neuroinflammatory disease of the nerve roots in your lumbar or sacral spine. Your physicians need to be informed of the results of this screening test as you need to obtain both a confirmatory diagnosis, and a treatment plan that is specific for your condition.

## 12. THE EQUIVOCAL OR INCONCLUSIVE MRI

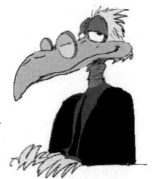

DR. BEAK says,
In equivocal cases,
medications that suppress
neuroinflammation should be
given a therapeutic trial.

AA is usually diagnosed on an axial MRI (foot to head) that shows cauda equina nerve root clumping that is adhered "glued" to the arachnoid lining (meninges) by adhesions. Prior to clumping and

[30]

adhering to the arachnoid lining, some nerve roots will enlarge (edema), displace, and present an asymmetrical picture. BE CLEARLY ADVISED: In the early phase of the development of AA, or in mild cases, some nerve roots may appear to cling together, enlarge, or displace, but they don't clearly form clumps or "glue" to the arachnoid lining. This can be a major problem in interpretation. "Is there early or mild clumping, or maybe not?"

The lateral (sagittal) MRI views in confirmed cases show such signs as thickened nerve roots, dilated lower spinal canal (thecal sac), spinal fluid flow obstruction, and leakage or seepage. The lateral view, however, is less precise and a diagnosis of AA is not usually possible solely on the lateral view.

What should be done in equivocal or marginal cases? We recommend a blood test for inflammatory markers and therapeutic trials with the potent anti-neuroinflammatory drugs ketorolac and methylprednisolone. If a person's pain and some other symptoms improve with the trial, AA is likely. The 3-component medical treatment for AA should then be instituted, providing the person has a typical history and physical findings of AA.

# 13. MOST COMMON CAUSE OF CONSTANT INCURABLE PAIN IS AA

It will probably surprise many people in this era of opioid controversy, but a lot of research has recently been done to identify the causes of constant incurable pain and develop treatments for it, which may require opioid medication.

Our studies show that the great majority (over 90%) of persons with constant incurable pain have one of only 6 underlying causes:

- ✓ Adhesive Arachnoiditis (AA)
- ✓ Genetic Collagen Disorders of the Ehlers-Danlos and Marfan Syndrome Types
- ✓ Reflex Sympathetic Dystrophy (RSD) - Chronic Regional Pain Syndrome (CRPS)
- ✓ Post-Stroke
- ✓ Traumatic Brain Injury (TBI)
- ✓ Autoimmune Disorders – Post Viral or Rheumatologic Type

# 14. I'VE BEEN DIAGNOSED WITH ADHESIVE ARACHNOIDITIS. NOW WHAT?

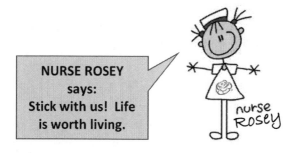

**NURSE ROSEY says:** Stick with us! Life is worth living.

nurse Rosey

Don't' panic. AA is now controllable in almost all cases. AA has traditionally been a diagnosis that brought great fear, since nothing could be done. NO MORE! There is now treatment that can allow greater function and pain relief than ever before! The sooner a treatment protocol is started, the better the potential outcome. It is important to have a "partner" in your care, be it a friend or family member, that can help you understand your disease and help you start a self-care program.

[32]

# 15. TWO STRATEGIES FOR TREATMENT

There are two major strategies of AA treatment: (1) medication to reduce neuroinflammation, promote neuroregeneration, and control pain; and (2) physiologic and preventive measures to enhance spinal fluid flow and prevent shrinkage of nerves, muscles, and collagen-based tissue.

| | | |
|---|---|---|
| **Medication to reduce neuroinflammation, promote neuroregeneration, and control pain.** |  | **Physiologic and preventive measures to improve spinal fluid flow and prevent tissue shrinkage.** |

The nerve roots of the cauda equina and the spinal canal covering (arachnoid and dura in the lower spine) are dependent upon spinal fluid flow to nourish and flush the spinal canal of toxins including neuroinflammatory waste. Since AA interferes with spinal fluid flow, people with AA must do daily simple physiologic measures to enhance spinal fluid flow such as: walking, arm and leg stretching, deep breathing, water soaking, or paraspinal massage. Other physiologic and preventive measures are to prevent shrinkage and scarring of nerves, muscle and supporting tissues that are either in or surround the spinal canal. For example, if the nerve roots of the cauda equina are not stretched, they may shrink which leads to bladder and bowel dysfunction, and possible partial leg paralysis. Most people with AA have some spinal fluid seepage into the tissues and muscles that run parallel to the spinal column. If these aren't stretched daily, they may shrink and prevent the arms from doing their normal extension and function. Some specific physiologic measures are designed to help reduce retained electricity which may form heat and inflammation. In summary every AA person needs an aggressive two-fold strategy of (1) medication; and (2) physiologic and preventive measures. It is our experience that people with AA may procrastinate and put off starting a two-fold strategy in hopes of a "single magic cure" or a physician who will come along and tell them exactly how to improve without the person and family developing their own two-fold strategy.

Here are the purposes and goals of the two-fold strategy:
1. Don't get worse
2. Maintain a quality of life
3. Achieve some permanent recovery

| MEDICATION | PHYSIOLOGIC AND PREVENTIVE MEASURES |
|---|---|
| ✓ Suppression of neuroinflammation | ✓ Prevent tissue and nerve shrinkage |
| ✓ Regrowth of damaged tissue (neuroregenesis) | ✓ Prevent impairment of legs, bladder, bowel (paralysis) |
| ✓ Pain control | ✓ Maintain body functions and a "LIFE" |

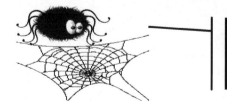

Happy Spider says, "No more paralysis or early death".

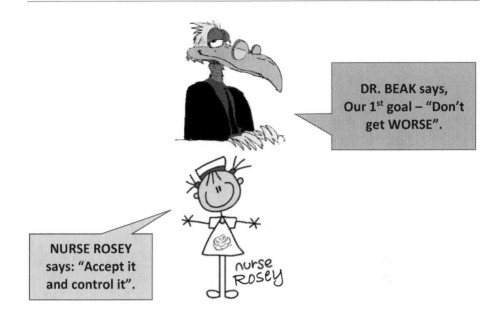

DR. BEAK says, Our 1st goal – "Don't get WORSE".

NURSE ROSEY says: "Accept it and control it".

# 16. MAJOR GOAL OF TREATMENT: STOP PROGRESSION - DON'T GET WORSE

The major goal of this handbook is to prevent people with AA from getting worse. We caution those who are in the mild or moderate categories against complacency. Neuroinflammation is the culprit of AA. If you don't constantly take measures to control it, for unknown reasons, it may flare and cause worsening in a short time period. In summary, once you have AA, as documented on an MRI, you must constantly take measures to control neuroinflammation lest you risk sudden and unexpected worsening.

AA is a neuroinflammatory disease of the nerve roots and the spinal canal covering. Once started, the neuroinflammation of AA may take any of these paths:

1. Total recovery or resolution (usually in mild or asymptomatic cases).
2. Cause progressive neurologic damage such as to involve the bladder, intestine, sex organs, or legs.
3. Go into periods of "false" remission only to episodically flare.

> **If you have AA, you should plan on being on an indefinite, dual strategy treatment program. If you choose to ignore possible progression, you can find yourself having sudden, without warning, neurologic impairments.**

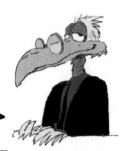

# 17. THE EARLIER THE TREATMENT—THE BETTER THE RESULT

Our conclusion in evaluating and treating several hundred AA cases is that the earlier treatment is started, the better the result or outcome.

> **This handbook is primarily designed to get you started – NOW!! Don't expect or wait for your doctors to tell you all you should know.**

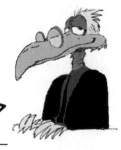

WHY?  NI causes adhesions to form between the cauda equina nerve roots and the arachnoid lining of the spinal canal.  In the early stage of AA, adhesions and NI can be at least partially resolved.  After a time, however, NI and adhesions can cause permanent nerve damage that is not resolvable.

# 18. THREE- COMPONENT MEDICAL TREATMENT

Our research and experience are clear.  Effective medical treatment requires a three-component medication program:

1.  Suppression of neuroinflammation;
2.  Regrowth of damaged nerve tissue (neuroregeneration)
3.  Pain control

The 3-components must be simultaneously administered. Unfortunately, only a limited number of drugs are effective in treating AA.  Drugs that help AA must cross the blood-brain barrier, enter the spinal fluid, and bind to action points (called receptors) on specific cells known as glia in the nerve roots of the cauda equina.

The proper treatment of confirmed cases of AA requires the simultaneous administration of these 3-components:

1.  Suppress Neuroinflammation
     Examples: ketorolac, methylprednisolone,
     acetazolamide
2.  Promote Damaged Nerve Regrowth (Neuroregeneration)
     Examples: pregnenolone, human chorionic
     gonadotropin (HCG), nandrolone
3.  Pain Control

Examples: low dose naltrexone, gabapentin, opioids, clonidine, ketamine

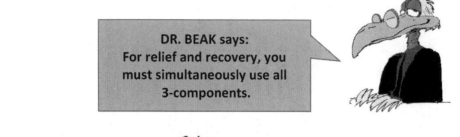

**DR. BEAK says:**
For relief and recovery, you must simultaneously use all 3-components.

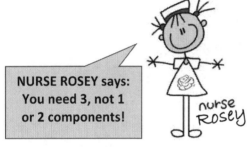

**NURSE ROSEY says:**
You need 3, not 1 or 2 components!

The amount of permanent recovery a person with AA can achieve, in our opinion, is related to the use of the neuroregeneration agents. These are hormones that reduce neuroinflammation and promote neuroregeneration.

Currently most physicians are not yet familiar with the 3-component protocol or treatment. It is no more complex or difficult than the multiple drug protocols necessary to treat such common diseases as asthma, emphysema, diabetes, or depression. The 3-component medical protocol we recommend can and should be done by medical providers in every community.

Out of over a dozen anti-inflammatory drugs on the commercial market, only ketorolac is consistently effective in AA. Sometimes diclofenac and indomethacin seem to help. Out of a dozen corticosteroids on the market, only methylprednisolone (Medrol®) and dexamethasone (Decadron®) are consistently effective. Although the menu of drugs isn't as extensive as we would like, there are enough drugs for a person to get started with AA treatment.

Pain control is what is usual in medical practice today. The drug naltrexone is the preferred pain reliever to start with, but it cannot be given to persons who currently take opioids since it will cause withdrawal symptoms. Many people with AA have constant pain "24/7" as opposed to intermittent "comes and goes" pain. Severe constant pain will usually require a nerve conduction agent such as gabapentin or topiramate to enhance nerve function.

Undoubtedly, new and better drugs will be identified as the list in this handbook is considered "first generation." Although better drugs are likely in the future, no person with AA should delay starting a 3-component medication program.

Currently, people with AA in the severe and catastrophic categories are typically those who have not had the opportunity to participate in 3-component medical treatment. To move from a severe or catastrophic category to a lesser category is not impossible as we have witnessed many people with AA accomplish this feat. Be advised that almost all have been on a 3-component treatment protocol, and have taken the nerve and tissue building hormones, human chorionic gonadotropin and/or nandrolone.

There are some physicians and on-lookers who claim there is no treatment for AA since the United States Food and Drug Administration (FDA) has not labeled a specific drug for AA treatment. Hopefully the future will bring about such labeling, but we seriously doubt that any one drug will do the job since AA is a complex disease.

# 19. NEUROINFLAMMATION AND NEURODEGENERATION

To treat AA and live a good life, you must clearly understand what these 2 terms mean – "neuroinflammation" and "neurodegeneration". Furthermore, you must know that these 2 conditions must be treated simultaneously to get improvement.

| NEUROINFLAMMATION | NEURODEGENERATION |
|---|---|
| AA can cause microglial cells in the spinal cord and nerve roots to inflame which is called neuroinflammation. | When deterioration and disintegration of nerve tissues is present the tissues become non-functional, and pain, impairment, and bizarre sensations occur. Tissue degeneration leads to autoimmunity |

| SOME ANTI-NEUROINFLAMMATION DRUGS | SOME NEUROREGENERATIVE DRUGS |
| --- | --- |
| Ketorolac, methylprednisolone, curcumin, metformin, acetazolamide, pentoxifylline | Nandrolone, human chorionic gonadotropin, dehydroepiandrosterone (DHEA), pregnenolone |

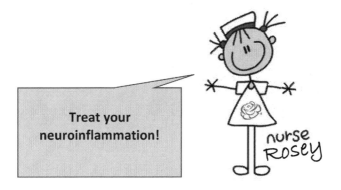

Treat your neuroinflammation!

nurse Rosey

Pain relief drugs such as opioids, gabapentin, and devices such as electrical stimulators provide temporary symptomatic relief. They do not provide long-term disease reduction which only occurs when neuroinflammatory and neuroregenerative drugs are taken.

ASK YOURSELF: Are you taking drugs to suppress neuroinflammation and promote neuroregeneration? If not, you should start because otherwise you can't expect to control AA, much less achieve some permanent recovery.

# 20. SEVEN FACTS ABOUT NEUROINFLAMMATION (NI)

Fact 1: The fundamental cause of AA is neuroinflammation. It must be controlled or the person with AA will be in severe pain, and will progressively deteriorate.

Fact 2: The term inflammation is a generic term that can apply to any tissue in the body due to any cause. Neuroinflammation is a specific and special type of inflammation caused by nerve cells called microglia, which are found in the spinal cord, brain, and nerve roots of the cauda equina.

Fact 3: Active neuroinflammation causes tissue destruction, adhesions, and fibrosis "scarring." This combination causes clumps or "hard lumps" inside the spinal canal so cerebral spinal fluid (CSF) flow is obstructed "blocked." CSF can also leak through the spinal canal covering into surrounding tissues causing further inflammation and damage. It may also progressively destroy cauda equina nerve root connections to your legs, bladder, sex organs, and bowel.

Fact 4: Neuroinflammation may be active and will silently, without awareness by the person, destroy nerve tissue.

Fact 5: The drugs that suppress the inflammation of arthritis, allergies, and asthma may not suppress neuroinflammation. Why? To suppress neuroinflammation, a drug must cross the blood-brain barrier and bind or attach to the microglial cell. Consequently, the number of drugs, that suppress neuroinflammation are few.

Fact 6: If you have found that ketorolac (Toradol®), or one of these corticosteroids, methylprednisolone (Medrol®), dexamethasone (Decadron®), provide pain and symptom relief, you have fundamentally demonstrated that you have active neuroinflammation that needs on-going treatment usually with one of these 2 agents.

Fact 7: Neuroinflammation may lead to autoimmune disorders that can manifest in other areas of the body. Some autoimmune manifestations are arthritis, thyroiditis, muscle pains, fatigue, and carpel tunnel syndrome.

The medical treatment suggested in this handbook cannot be guaranteed as far as outcome. By use of the 3-component medication program however, few persons in our experience worsen, because it is primarily geared toward suppression of neuroinflammation and promotion of neuroregeneration. Some people with AA have found a "near-cure" with the 3-component program. We are hesitant to use the term "cure" as neuroinflammation may remain asymptomatic and re-emerge later. Once AA is observed on an MRI, treatment must likely be a lifetime endeavor.

# 21. PHYSIOLOGIC TREATMENT MEASURES

Physiologic measures have 3 major goals:
1. Enhance spinal fluid flow
2. Reduce neuroinflammation,
3. Prevent tissue shrinkage and paralysis.

While it may not be necessary to do every measure, every AA person should do some of the following every day.

- ✓ Walking with arm swings
- ✓ Water soaking including foot baths
- ✓ Deep breathing and breath holding
- ✓ Rocking chair or swing
- ✓ Trampoline walking
- ✓ Stretching – side-to-side, arm and leg extension
- ✓ Magnet rubs
- ✓ Copper jewelry
- ✓ Sing or whistle

When our AA research and education project began 10 years ago it was common to see people with AA who had partial paralysis "paraparesis" of the legs and arms. In some cases, the paralysis was so bad that the person had to use a wheelchair or was confined to bed. Many people could not raise their arms or legs to their full extension. Unfortunately, about the only treatment these people ever had was pain medication. Until recently there was no knowledge about spinal fluid flow, leakage and seepage, tissue shrinking, and retained electricity. In recent years as treatment of neuroinflammation and specialized physiologic measures have become known, we see few new people with AA who have paralysis of the legs and/or a diminution of arm extension.

Here are reasons and some specific physiologic measures:

Increase Spinal Fluid Flow: deep breathing, walking, stand and stretch arms, sing and/or whistle, rock in a rocking chair or swing, walk on a trampoline

Prevention of Tissue Shrinkage and Scarring: walking, side-to-side stretching, extend legs, arms, and feet

Elimination of Inflammation and Electricity: water soaking, foot baths, wearing copper jewelry, magnet rubs, massage

# 22. PREVENTIVE MEASURES TO "NOT GET WORSE"

The very criteria of an MRI diagnosis of AA means one has nerve clumping with adhesions. This indicates that there is already neuroinflammation and nerve damage INSIDE the spinal canal. When AA is seen on an MRI, goal number one is to "not get worse." Our recommended strategy for treatment of AA is two-fold: (1) medication; (2) physiologic and preventive measures. Here is a list of simple preventive measures for everyday practice to "not get worse."

1. Use bench type chairs/seats (avoid bucket type seats)
2. Posture – sit straight up and walk "straight up"

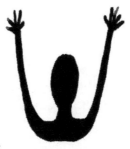

3. Swing arms when walking_____
4. Supportive footwear. No thongs, open heel, or high heel shoes. Make sure sandals have heel/ankle straps.
5. Wear a copper bracelet or anklet
6. Deep breath a few times every couple of hours
7. Stretch arms, legs, and hips each day
8. Take walks twice a day

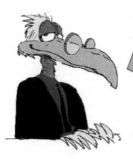

DR. BEAK says: Preventive measures help to improve spinal fluid flow, avoid paralysis, and prevent impairment of bladder and other organs.

9. Soak in a tub of water. Daily is best. If no tub, jacuzzi, or pool, take a long shower
10. Use an electromagnetic or microcurrent electric device, 3 to 5 times a week (infrared, laser, radio wave)
11. Wear a brace when taking a long automobile or plane ride
12. Don't sit in one position for more than 45 minutes

[46]

13. Don't lift over 10-15 pounds
14. Don't exhaust yourself or do activities that cause pain

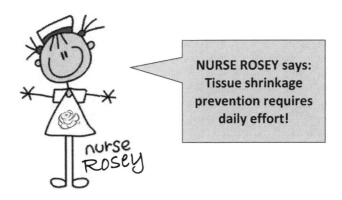

NURSE ROSEY says:
Tissue shrinkage
prevention requires
daily effort!

nurse
Rosey

# 23. SPINAL FLUID – RIVER OF HOPE!!

Optimal function and movement of spinal fluid flow is critical to the relief and recovery of people with AA.

How is it made?

Spinal fluid is made from arterial blood in a structure in the brain called the choroid plexus. Cells with fine structure called cilia and micro-villi strain and produce CSF in the brain. About 125 ml of fluid is produced every 4 to 6 hours for a daily total of about 500 ml.

How does it flow?

Once made, spinal fluid travels like a river around the brain and down the spinal canal. Once it reaches the bottom (lumbar-sacral) area, it flows back up the spinal canal to be filtered by lymph nodes in the neck. Once impurities are removed in the lymph nodes, spinal fluid is pumped into the blood stream to be excreted out of the body by urination. Deep breathing and arm swings helps the spinal fluid flow.

## What does spinal fluid do?

1. Carries nutrients and the body's natural healing elements to the brain, spinal cord and cauda equina nerve roots

2. Lubricates and protects the brain, spinal cord, and cauda equina from developing friction, neuroinflammation, and adhesions

3. Carries out toxins (e.g. inflammatory waste)

The clumping of nerve roots and the formation of adhesions cause disruption and obstruction of spinal fluid flow. This is like putting large rocks or a dam in a river – the water flow will slow down, back up, or reroute around the blockage.

When blockage occurs inside the spinal canal symptoms of headache, blurred vision, nausea, dizziness, mental confusion, loss of memory, ringing in ears, loss of balance, dysphoria (opposite of euphoria), vertigo and fatigue may occur.

One medication that often reduces the symptoms of spinal fluid flow obstruction is acetazolamide, given 50 to 500 mg a day. Our suggestion is to start at about 50 mg a day and work up the dosage to 250 mg a day over 2 weeks. Stop if it's not helping. Continue and even raise the dosage if acetazolamide helps. This drug also reduces neuroinflammation. Every person with AA should consider it.

[48]

# 24. SPINAL FLUID LEAKAGE AND SEEPAGE

> The "rusty", seeping "pipe"

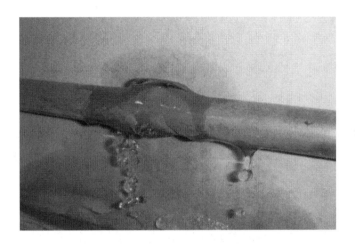

We have learned from MRI reviews and physical examinations most people with AA chronically leak or "seep" spinal fluid into the tissues between the lumbar spine area and skin over the area. The process resembles a pipe that rusts and chronically leaks or "seeps" fluids out of the pipe. Unfortunately, the formation of inflammation between the nerve roots and arachnoid lining may cause microleaks through the outer spinal canal covering.

The Problem

Spinal fluid is toxic to muscle, subcutaneous fat, and skin which is why spinal fluid is in a closed canal away from non-CNS tissue. The exposure of spinal fluid to the general circulation may also cause an autoimmune disorder.

[49]

Spinal fluid that leaks into the tissues between the spinal column and skin over the lumbar spine area is toxic to these tissues. It will cause inflammation, scarring, and shrinkage of muscles, fascia, nerves and skin.

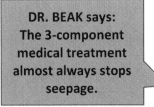
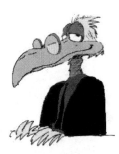

DR. BEAK says:
The 3-component
medical treatment
almost always stops
seepage.

## Symptoms and Complications

Pain and indentation of the skin along the spine may occur. A major complication is that muscles and nerves that run along the spinal column may shrink and decrease one's ability to fully extend the arms and legs.

## Diagnosis

Active "seepage" is suspected if there is pain upon pressing on the skin and tissues over the lumbar spine. If a topical skin anesthetic such as lidocaine relieves pain, seepage is likely. Seepage evidence can be seen on MRI.

Over-time, these complications from spinal fluid seepage may occur:

1. Shrinkage of paraspinal muscles to the point that you can't fully extend your arms or legs.
2. Pain over the spine – worse when pressure is applied.
3. Abnormal, off-balance leaning – asymmetry of back muscles.
4. Indentation (caving in) of tissues over the spine.

# 25. HOW TO IMPROVE YOUR SPINAL FLUID FLOW

All people with AA will have some disruption or blockage of spinal fluid flow. Good spinal fluid flow is necessary to wash away waste products and bring nutrition and healing power to the inflamed site.

Here are simple physiologic measures to enhance spinal fluid flow. We recommend daily use of at least some of them.

- ✓ Rock in a rocking chair or swing
- ✓ Walk on a trampoline
- ✓ Use vibrator or massager over spine (Back scratchers and scrubbers are good)
- ✓ Soak or wade in water or use foot baths
- ✓ Walk and swing your arms "Power Walking"
- ✓ Rock back and forth on your feet
- ✓ Rub your spine with copper and/or a magnet
- ✓ Nod your head up and down
- ✓ Scrub your back with a brush
- ✓ Deep breathing (diaphragm) with stomach

# 26. TREATMENT OF SPINAL FLUID LEAKAGE AND SEEPAGE

If seepage is present it can almost always be seen on your MRI. Above all else, you need to be on a 3-component medical treatment program for AA:

1.  Suppression of neuroinflammation
2.  Promotion of neuroregenesis
3.  Pain control

Here are some other measures used to stop spinal fluid leakage and seepage:

- Add an anti-inflammatory or neuroregenerative agent to the current treatment program
- Massage into the lumbar area a topical cream which contains a corticosteroid like prednisone.
- Inject a corticoid and/or homeopathic agent into the tissue around (not in) the spinal column.

SPECIAL NOTES

1.  We believe spinal fluid leaks regularly stop with the neuroinflammatory and neuroregeneration agents suggested in this handbook.

2. We do not recommend blood patches since they are for acute and not the chronic leakage present in persons with AA

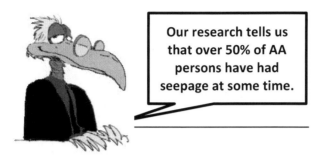

# 27. STRETCHES TO PREVENT TISSUE SHRINKAGE

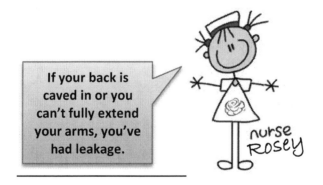

<u>Stretching Principals</u>

1. Stretch to a point you feel tugging or pulling but not pain
2. Standing is best to stretch but sitting or lying down is OK
3. Stretch your arms and legs into positions that let you know you are tugging or pulling on your lumbar area

It is the shrinking, scarring, and shortening of nerves, muscle, and tendons that cause severe neurologic impairments such as partial paralysis "paraparesis." The nerve roots of the cauda equina are the first section of long nerves "e.g. sciatic nerve" that reach into your legs, feet, bladder, intestine, stomach, rectum/anus, and sex organs.

Muscles and tendons that attach to the vertebrae and joints can also shrink, particularly with chronic spinal fluid seepage.

Here are simple stretching exercises to prevent tissue shrinkage.

1 – Reach for the sky. Spread your fingers, raise both arms straight up. Hold for 5 to 10 seconds. Raise only as high as you can without causing pain.

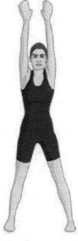

2 – Side to side bends. Stand with hands on head. Lean right for 5 to 10 seconds, then left for 5 to 10 seconds. Bend only right and left to feel a "tug" or "pressure" in your lower back, but not pain.

[54]

NURSE ROSEY says: These exercises help spinal fluid flow and prevent tissue shrinkage.

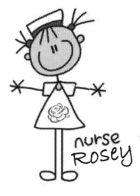

nurse Rosey

## Other Helpful Stretching Exercises

Full-Body Stretch Laying Down: Lay down on a flat surface (if physically possible) and do a full-body stretch with arms over head. Count to 10.

Sit and Stretch Arms: Stretch your arms and spread your fingers. Count to 10. Can do while sitting in a car or plane.

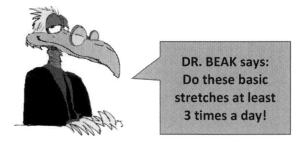

DR. BEAK says: Do these basic stretches at least 3 times a day!

Leg Raise While Laying Down: Raise each leg until you feel tugging in your back. Count to 10.

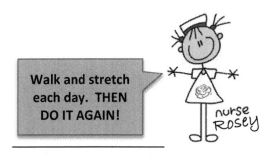

**Walk and stretch each day. THEN DO IT AGAIN!**

nurse Rosey

<u>Leg Raise While Standing:</u> Stabilize yourself next to a table or wall. Raise your leg and flex your foot. Count to 10.

<u>Knee Pull While Laying Down</u>: Pull one knee back until you feel tugging in your back. Count to 10. Repeat with the other knee.

## 28. WALKING WITH ARM SWINGS: THE BEST EXERCISE

A person with AA **must take walks every day** to move spinal fluid and prevent shrinking of nerves and muscles. Walk with toes pointed straight ahead. Swing your arms during part of your walk. Lift your head so that your ears are directly over your shoulders. Breathe deeply. Quit at the first feeling of fatigue. Don't overdo or push too hard.

People with AA should wear supportive, tie shoes such as tennis shoes unless tie shoes, cause pain. There are also some shoes that have copper or magnets in the soles. These are excellent to help control pain.

Bare foot is often better for people with AA than the modern-day practice of wearing thongs, sandals, flip flops, or slip-ons. Non-supportive footwear is a risk in 2 ways: (1) falls; (2) prevents walking with correct posture.

One slip, slide, or fall can set a person with AA back to square one or worse. A fall may tear adhesions which may cause severe pain and healing with more permanent, nerve entrapments and impairments!

# 29. RETAINED ELECTRICITY – MUST ELIMINATE

Nerves function and control our body's organs and structures by transmitting electricity. With AA, nerve roots are clumped with adhesions and scarring so electricity won't pass easily up or down the nerve root. Consequently, electricity is retained and accumulates.

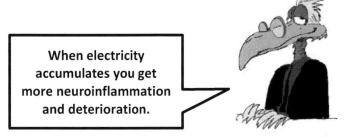

**When electricity accumulates you get more neuroinflammation and deterioration.**

When electricity accumulates, it causes increased neuroinflammation and it may suddenly release itself in dysfunctional bursts. That is why a person with AA gets:

- ✓ Shooting and burning episodes of pain
- ✓ Leg jerks and tremors

Abnormal electricity retention and release also contributes to such symptoms as burning feet and funny sensations on skin such as "bugs crawling" and "water dripping."

Here are physiologic measures to eliminate electricity.  Do some daily:

- ✓ Rub your spine with copper or a magnet 2 to 3 times a day
- ✓ Wear a copper anklet or bracelet
- ✓ Use magnets in your shoes or mattress
- ✓ Wear lots of jewelry, particularly copper
- ✓ Hold doorknobs or other metal a second longer
- ✓ Soak in water and foot baths (Epsom salts help)
- ✓ Pet your dog or cat (any fur will do.)
- ✓ Walk barefoot on carpet or outside on your lawn

# 30. YOU NEED MORE OXYGEN

Oxygen is necessary for healing, nerve function, and medication effectiveness.  Without enough, you may progressively deteriorate.

<u>Symptoms of Low Oxygen</u>

- Fatigue and Lethargy
- Slow or Forgetful Thinking
- Depression and Feeling of Hopelessness

- Tired, But Can't Sleep
- Pain Medication Works Poorly
- Deep sighing

How Do I Get Oxygen?

Oxygen is breathed in through your lungs and enters your blood stream to be carried throughout your body. Whether your pain site is in the spine, brain, joints, or muscles, you must have oxygen for pain relief and healing. The more oxygen, the better.

How Do I Get More Oxygen?

Your base oxygen intake and carrying capacity is what is in your blood when you are quietly sitting or lying down. Anytime you become active you breathe a little harder and deeper and your heart pumps a little faster, so you carry more oxygen in your blood. The healing and pain relief formula is simply to stay more active than what you are when you sit or lay down. Just increasing your breathing and heart rate will increase oxygen at your pain site.

1. Stay active! Walk every day.
2. Breathe as deeply as you can with your stomach (diaphragm) and hold it for a few seconds. Do it while sitting or standing. Do it in a car, church, or at home. Do this at least 10 times a day.

# 31. A NEW BREAKTHROUGH: ELECTROMAGNETIC THERAPY

A new therapy that is gaining more and more supporters and advocates is electromagnetic energy (EME) therapy. We highly recommend it as we believe EME enhances the standard treatments of medicinal agents and physiologic measures.

[59]

Human beings are alive and functioning because cells metabolize and communicate with each other by electromagnetic energy (EME). EME is biologically ½ magnetism and ½ electricity and the devices administer it in waves. Devices that "pulse" or administer the energy in "waves" are most effective.

EME Devices: There are 3 medical devices that administer EME in various wave lengths and frequency to obtain a clinical effect:

1. Radio waves that are deep, long waves of slow frequency (Provant®)
2. Infrared has shallow warm waves
3. Laser has deep, short, and hot waves of high frequency

## Difference with Other Devices

✓ TENS and electrical stimulators provide pure electricity which may provide temporary pain relief. Microcurrents are particularly effective for pain relief
✓ Acupuncture –moves retained electricity, unblocks and opens energy channels to enhance healing

## Benefits of EME

EME reduces inflammation, edema, and retained electricity; These devices have been shown to have considerable healing power unless the tissue is scarred and non-functional.

[60]

We believe EME devices are helpful to heal spinal fluid leakage and even promote neuroregeneration in some cases. At this point in time we recommend a one-month trial of EME to see if a positive clinical effect can be obtained. To date, about 2/3 of people with AA report a positive benefit in pain reduction and functional improvement. We also recommend electric devices. In summary, all people with AA should be on the 3-componant medication program accompanied by physiologic measures. Once in place, all people with AA should explore the use of EME and electrical devices.

# 32. THE IMPORTANCE OF SPINE BRACING

People with AA must be very cautious and careful while lifting, bending over, or walking in an unfamiliar area. If you attempt to lift something that weighs more than about 10-15 pounds, you run the risk of tearing adhesions or scars in and around your lower spinal canal. When you bend over, raise up slowly because a jerk or rapid movement can cause a tear or rip. If this happens, severe pain follows, and the damaged area may end up being worse than ever.

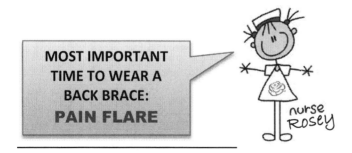

MOST IMPORTANT
TIME TO WEAR A
BACK BRACE:
PAIN FLARE

nurse
Rosey

People with AA need to wear a brace to protect their damaged area in these circumstances.

<u>Worst Situation</u>: Riding in a car or plane that has bucket seats.

<u>Danger Situation</u>: Walking in unfamiliar areas such as a shopping center, grocery store, or social event.

# 33. DO YOU HAVE A GENETIC COLLAGEN DISORDER LIKE EHLERS-DANLOS SYNDROME (EDS)?

AA occurs frequently in persons who have a genetic collagen disorder of which Ehlers-Danlos Syndrome (EDS) and Marfan Syndrome are the most common. These genetic disorders have a built-in gene that prevents soft (non-bone) tissues from being formed properly during embryogenesis. As a person grows into childhood and adulthood this gene defect causes tissue to progressively deteriorate, degenerate, and form micro-tears in tissue. Tissues most affected are those that are known as "connective" in that they support and connect such organs as the intestine, joints, skin, blood vessels, and spinal cord to bones and fibrous tissue. Fundamentally, the disorder causes tissue to stretch, loosen, and collapse due to the dissolution of collagen. Unfortunately, the spinal canal has many soft connective tissues like the pia mater and arachnoid. They may collapse and cause an array of spinal conditions such as Chiari malformations, Tarlov Cysts, tethered cord, syringomyelia, and AA.

<u>Test yourself with these questions to see if you may have a genetic collagen disorder.</u>

1. Has anyone in your family had Ehlers-Danlos Syndrome, Marfan Syndrome, or a ruptured organ or aneurysm?

2. Have you developed a sudden, without warning or trauma, a loss or impairment of a neurologic function such as lifting or flexing your arms and legs, urination, or had a ruptured organ or aneurysm?

3. Have you had multiple teeth totally deteriorate or fall out?

4. Have you developed a sudden, constant pain in one spot on your body without warning or trauma?

5. Do you have deformities of your hands or feet?

6. Can you now (or could you ever) do a forward bend and place your hands flat on the floor without bending your knees?

7. Can you now (or could you ever) bend your thumb to touch your forearm?

8. As a child did you amuse your friends by contorting your body into strange shapes or could you do the splits?

9. As a child or teenager did your shoulder or kneecap dislocate on more than one occasion?

10. Do you consider yourself double-jointed?

11. Does your skin easily break, tear, crack, or bruise?

If you answered yes to 4 or more of these questions, your physician should evaluate you for the presence of a genetic collagen disorder of which the best known are called "Ehlers-Danlos and Marfan Syndromes."

# 34. COLLAGEN BUILDING PROGRAM FOR PEOPLE WITH AA AND GCD

People with genetic collagen disorders (GCD), of which Ehlers-Danlos Syndrome (EDS), and Marfan Syndromes are the best known, frequently develop AA and other neurologic complications such as Tarlov Cysts, Chiari malformations/herniations, tethered cord, and syringomyelia among others.

> Our research and experience are clear. When you have the dual diseases of AA and GCD, you must be treated with the 3-component medical protocol - **PLUS** – You must take measures to build collagen, **BOTH INSIDE AND OUTSIDE** of the CNS.

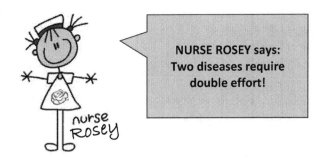

NURSE ROSEY says:
Two diseases require
double effort!

nurse
Rosey

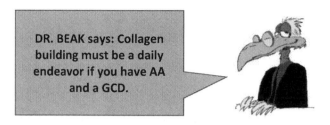

DR. BEAK says: Collagen building must be a daily endeavor if you have AA and a GCD.

RATIONALE: Persons with GCD's are genetically programmed at birth to build faulty collagen which causes tissue to dissolve and break down easily in their "connective" tissues that hold organs in place. Some persons start to dissolve tissues in childhood and others in adulthood. Tissues in the spine, eye, gums, and brain such as the pia mater and arachnoid are made of collagen. A person with AA and a GCD must constantly attempt to build collagen to combat its dissolution.

<u>Here are our Collagen Building Measures for Dual Diseases</u>

| DIET & DIETARY SUPPLEMENTS | EXERCISES | NON-PRESCRIPTION HORMONES | PRESCRIPTION HORMONES |
|---|---|---|---|
| High Protein Diet<br><br>DIETARY SUPPLEMENTS<br>Collagen (gummies, powder, liquid), Bone Broth, Vitamin $B_{12}$, C, Magnesium | Light Weightlifting<br><br>Walking<br><br>Mild Stretching | Colostrum<br><br>Gonadal Extract (Orchex®, or other)<br><br>Deer Antler Velvet | Human Chorionic Gonadotropin: 250-500 units, 3 times a week<br><br>and/or<br><br>Nandrolone Troche: 25mg, 1 a day on 3-5 days a week or injection, 25-50mg, once a week |

# 35. INSOMNIA AND SLEEP

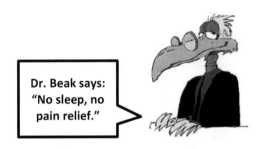

A regular sleep pattern enhances the hormone and immunologic systems that are necessary for healing and neuroregeneration.  Here are some guidelines:

✓ Be in bed between 10:00 and 11:30 PM
✓ Perform your last stretches and take your medications 30 to 60 minutes before bedtime
✓ Keep your pain medications beside your bed.  Take additional dosages during the night, if necessary
✓ Take your first morning pain relief medications so you can be out of bed between 6:00 and 8:00 AM
✓ Goal is 4 to 8 sleeping hours each night.  Do not expect more than four hours of consecutive sleep
✓ If a sleep aid is needed, we recommend clonidine, gabapentin, melatonin, valerian root, or temazepam

[66]

# 36. HIGH PROTEIN ANTI-INFLAMMATORY DIET

Our recommended diet is principally based on the physiological fact that amino acids and collagen build tissue. It is designed to help reduce neuroinflammation and promote healing.

Although much has been written and proclaimed about various diets for pain control, hard evidence that they really contribute is lacking. Our experience, however, is that people with AA who follow a high protein, anti-inflammatory diet, do better than the average person.

THE DIET

Protein Food: red meat, pork, poultry, fish, eggs, soy, dairy products, cottage cheese. If you can't or won't eat any of these, you must obtain protein powder drinks and/or protein bars.

Collagen/Amino Acid Preparations: To help build tissue take collagen or amino acid preparations every day. Collagen gummies, capsules, liquid powder, amino acid capsules, liquid, powders. (See label for instructions.)

Vegetables and Fruits: Some vegetables and fruits have anti-inflammatory properties. Eat one or more of these each day.

| Carrot | Celery | Avocado | Tomatoes |
| Broccoli | Onion | Dark Leafy Greens | Cucumbers |
| Radish | Berries | Apple | Citrus |
| Beets | | | |

Drinks: (Only use dietary sugars if weight is a problem): Coffee, Tea, Dietary Drinks, Water, Low alcohol content drinks are acceptable.

Banned to Control Weight:  Milk, Regular Sodas, Fruit Juice, Bread

Highly Restricted to Control Weight: (Eat these very sparingly):
Potatoes, Corn, Cakes/Pies, Pasta/Pizza, ice cream, whipping cream

Gluten Restriction: bread, pasta, rolls, noodles (For some avoiding gluten helps digestion)

Dietary Supplements: Pick some for weekly use
Co-Enzyme Q-10
Omega 3 Fish Oil
Vitamins:  C, D, $B_{12,}$ $B_6$
Minerals:  Calcium and Magnesium
Probiotic

# 37. INVERSION THERAPY

Inversion therapy (IT) is a form of super-stretching.  It is usually done on a commercial stretcher.  Some people with AA hang upside down as a therapy.  The purpose of IT is to stretch out nerves, muscles, and tendons that have shrunk or are about to shrink.  This is especially a problem with persons who have had spinal fluid leakage.  It must be done gently and for only a short time (e.g. 3 to 5 minutes) to begin.  Later, stretch time can be extended.  Only some people with AA seem to benefit from IT.  Those persons who can't fully extend their arms or legs are the best candidates.  We only recommend IT for persons who are on a 3-component medication program.  IT is an ancillary measure and not a primary treatment.

CAUTION:  Only stretch to the point of pressure.  <u>NEVER</u> cause pain because pain means you may be tearing tissue that may later scar, shrink, and produce even more pain.

DANGER:  Not to be done by people with AA who have heart disease or GCD.

# 38. AUTOIMMUNITY WITH AA

It is known that neither spinal fluid nor spinal cord tissue should get outside the spinal canal.  Why?  They are toxic to the general circulation and may cause an autoimmune disorder if too much spinal fluid or tissue gets out.  In AA, leakage or seepage of fluid into the tissues surrounding the spinal canal is a potential autoimmune trigger. So are tissue fragments from neuroinflammation that reach the general circulation through the normal spinal fluid cleansing mechanism in the brain and lymph nodes in the neck.

The presence of an autoimmune disorder becomes known to the person and medical practitioner when the person with AA begins to develop aches and pains in joints and muscles which are anatomically far away from the lumbar spine.  Some common autoimmune manifestations that may occur are Hashimoto's thyroiditis, carpal tunnel (and other nerve entrapments), temporal mandibular joint disease, and migraines. Food, smell and medication sensitivities can develop.  The most ominous sign of an out-of-control autoimmune disorder is tissue wasting, loss of appetite, weight loss, and susceptibility to infections.  This "wasting" state calls for tissue building hormones such as testosterone, human chorionic gonadotropin (HCG), or nandrolone.

# 39. STEM CELLS, MICROSURGERY, AND OTHER NEW PROCEDURES

People with AA may be consistently bombarded with offers to try experimental or expensive procedures. While we are aware of anecdotal, positive results with some of these treatments, we are also aware of reports of no effect or even worsening of AA. We believe all AA persons must initially be treated with a medical program consisting of 3 components:

1. Suppression of neuroinflammation
2. Regrowth of damaged nerves (neuroregeneration)
3. Pain control

Once a person with AA is on a 3-component medical treatment, a trial of stem cells, microsurgery, or other expensive or high-risk techniques are options if the person knows the risk.

Before any person with AA attempts a medical treatment outside the 3 basic medical components of treatment, discuss it with your family, other people with AA, and your primary medical practitioner.

There is not a day that goes by that we don't get asked, "What do you think about this or that new treatment?" The most common inquiries today involve stem cells. Here is our current view.

[70]

<u>Stem Cells</u>: An exciting development. Many techniques are being used under this broad title. In addition to cells, some non-cellular substrates that mimic or activate your own stem cells (e.g. laminins, amniotic fluid) are being tried. To date we have received mixed (some good, some worthless) reports on effectiveness, but none have reported any harm from any of the various stem cell therapies. Also, we have not received enough positive reports to **highly** recommend the treatment.

Any person with AA who tries a stem cell treatment is on their own for expense, risk, and benefit as experience with stem cells is still very meager.

<u>Microsurgery</u>: Not recommended at this time.

# 40. THERAPEUTIC TRIALS – FIND OUT WHAT WORKS

No two people with AA will likely have the same precise medical program. You must find your own "suit of clothes." We recommend a trial of 10 to 20 days of most medications as this is a long enough period to find out if a medication will work. Essentially every medication in the 3-component medical protocol can be given a 10 to 20-day trial. After that time, you will know if the drug causes side-effects or has a positive effect on pain, function, energy, or well-being.

Therapeutic trials with ketorolac, methylprednisolone (Medrol®), or dexamethasone (Decadron®) are highly recommended as they indicate whether neuroinflammation is at a high or low level. If you do a trial with one of these drugs and you feel much better, continue it on a low, intermittent dosage on 2 to 3 days a week. If a drug produces no positive effects after 10-20 days, there is no reason to continue it.

Common questions we get are: (1) Do I have AA? (2) If I have it, what do I do now? and (3) Why has my pain control stopped working? A therapeutic trial is used to find answers to these questions. If you relate to one of the above 3 questions, you are a candidate for therapeutic trials with ketorolac (Toradol®) and methylprednisolone (Medrol®).

We have found that ketorolac (Toradol®) and methylprednisolone (Medrol®) to be the most consistent agents to control neuroinflammation and treat AA. Unfortunately, many doctors and people with AA have erroneously been led to believe that these two drugs are too dangerous to use. Any party who believes this should re-evaluate their opinion due to new research and clinical experience.

---

**RISK vs BENEFIT**

**The risk vs benefit of developing serious complication of AA is greater than the risk of Toradol® and Medrol® if these 2 drugs are used as we suggest.**

---

# 41. HOW TO SAFELY TAKE KETOROLAC AND METHYLPREDNISOLONE

Ketorolac Trial: Take an injection or troche of 30 to 60 mg on 2 consecutive days.

[72]

### Safety Measures with Ketorolac (Toradol®)

a. Never use oral Toradol®
b. Use Toradol® as a compounded troche or as a commercially manufactured injection. Inject into buttocks.
c. Take blood urea nitrogen (BUN) and creatinine blood tests every 6 to 12 weeks if the person is high risk for kidney disease. High risk persons have diabetes, one kidney, or are over 70 years of age.

Methylprednisolone Trial: Take a 6-Day Dose Pak (Medrol® is the Trade Name)

Both Toradol® (30 to 60 mg) and Medrol® (2 to 4 mg) should only be taken maximally on 2 to 3 days a week. On this basis the risk is limited. The key to safety is to skip days between dosages.

# 42. PAIN CONTROL

BE CLEARLY ADVISED. New research clearly shows that there are three types of pain you must treat, if you have constant "24/7" pain. This table lists the 3 types of pain, cause, and some treatment agents.

| | |
|---|---|
| **1. NEUROINFLAMMATORY** | Due to inflammation in your cauda equina nerve roots and in the arachnoid lining of the spinal canal |
| Common treatment agents: ketorolac, Medrol®, acetazolamide, metformin, curcumin, indomethacin, low dose naltrexone (LDN), oxytocin, ketamine, opioids | |
| **2. NEUROPATHIC** | Due to nerve tissue (neurons, nerve roots, spinal cord) that has been damaged but is not inflamed |

| Common treatment agents: gabapentin, topiramate, clonazepam, carisoprodol, clonidine, diazepam | |
| --- | --- |
| **3. CENTRAL ELECTRICAL "Descending"** | Pain that is centralized and sends out aberrant electricity |
| Common treatment agents: Adderal®, methylphenidate, phentermine, modafinil, tizanidine | |

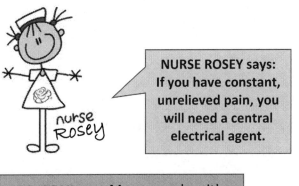

**NURSE ROSEY says:** If you have constant, unrelieved pain, you will need a central electrical agent.

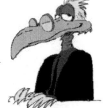

**DR. BEAK says:** Many people with AA have all 3 types of pain and must take a medication for each type.

# 43. BEST TREATMENT DRUGS FOR AA

Our research has found 7 drugs to be the most consistently effective in controlling AA. They are listed here. Other drugs help many individuals, but these shown here have been consistently effective in about 70-80% of people with AA.  You would be well-advised to show this list to your medical providers.

| Most consistent drugs to date: |
| --- |

| NEUROINFLAMMATION SUPPRESSORS |
| --- |
| Low Dose Naltrexone |
| Ketorolac |
| Methylprednisolone |
| Dexamethasone |
| Acetazolamide |
| **NERVE REGROWTH AGENTS "NEUROREGENERATION"** |
| Human Chorionic Gonadotropin |
| Nandrolone |

# 44. PROTOCOL FOR EMERGENCY TREATMENT OF SUSPECTED AA

Indication:  A person who has these SYMPTOMS within about 60 days after an epidural injection, spinal tap, or spine surgery.

Lumbar pain plus 2 of these symptoms:

1.  Burning/painful feet
2.  Bladder hesitancy/difficult to empty, can't hold urine
3.  Can't sit or stand in one place over 10 minutes
4.  Headache
5.  Blurred vision

6.  Leg pains

> **Any person who has had a spinal tap, epidural injection, or spine surgery and later experiences severe pain and some other neurologic symptoms, is a candidate for emergency AA treatment.**

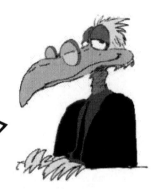

Treatment:

1.  6-day methylprednisolone, (Medrol®) dose pack
2.  Ketorolac (Toradol®) – 30 – 60 mg injection, daily for 2 or 3 days

Interpretation

If the person's pain and some other symptoms improve during the treatment, a diagnosis of early AA, cauda equina inflammation, or other CNS neuroinflammatory process has essentially been established. If, during or at the end of emergency treatment clinical improvement is apparent, we recommend the use of the 3-component medical protocol. If no improvement occurs, the logical conclusion is that pain and other symptoms are primarily non-inflammatory.

# 45. LOW DOSE NALTREXONE (LDN) FOR ADHESIVE ARACHNOIDITIS (AA)

About 75% of people with AA who have taken LDN have done well with it. Some people with AA in the mild and moderate categories even appear to be achieving almost a full recovery. Some are able to go about their pre-AA daily activities without much pain or impairment of body functions.

<u>Why Does LDN Work?</u>

Neuroinflammation is a major cause of pain. LDN is a potent neuroinflammation suppressor. LDN also activates the nervous system's pain centers that provide pain relief. You get two AA fighting actions with one drug.

<u>Dosage</u>

Dosage of LDN ranges from 0.5 to 5.0 mg a day. Most persons start at 0.5 or 1.0 mg and work up. Persons usually take LDN on 5 to 7 days a week. A compounding pharmacy can make LDN capsules, usually for a low monthly cost.

> **<u>IMPORTANT TREATMENT LIMITATION</u>**
> **Persons on DAILY opioid drugs CANNOT take LDN, because it will cause withdrawal symptoms.**

<u>Adding LDN to Your Current Treatment Protocol</u>

You can add LDN to your current protocol if you are not on opioids. (Some people on low dose opioids can also take LDN.) LDN can be taken with other anti-neuroinflammatory and neuroregeneration drugs including ketorolac, methylprednisolone, and all other non-opioid agents recommended in the 3-component protocol.

Suggestion: All people with AA NOT ON HIGH DOSE OPIOIDS should give LDN a 2to 4-week trial. You will know in this time frame whether it is helping you. A few people can have increased pain or have other side effects with LDN and cannot take it.

# 46. DRUGS IN THE 3 MEDICATION COMPONENTS

Only a few drugs effectively suppress neuroinflammation, promote neuroregenesis (nerve regrowth), and control the pain of AA. Why? To be effective a drug must cross the blood brain barrier, enter the spinal fluid, and attach to receptors on cauda equina nerve roots and glial cells. Shown in the following table are drugs reported to us by people with AA to be effective.

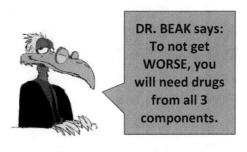

DR. BEAK says: To not get WORSE, you will need drugs from all 3 components.

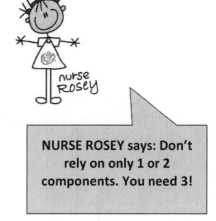

NURSE ROSEY says: Don't rely on only 1 or 2 components. You need 3!

[78]

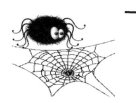

Happy Spider says:
Non-Prescription drugs
will boost your regular
prescriptions drugs.

| COMPONENT NO 1 | COMPONENT NO 2 | COMPONENT NO 3 |
|---|---|---|
| SUPRESSION OF NEUROINFLAMMATION | NEUROGENERATION (RE-GROWTH OF DAMAGED NERVES) | PAIN CONTROL |
| **Prescription drugs** | **Prescription drugs** | **Prescription drugs** |
| methylprednisolone (Medrol®), ketorolac, dexamethasone, metformin, acetazolamide, minocycline, indomethacin | human chorionic gonadotropin, nandrolone, testosterone, medroxyprogesterone | **General Agents:** naltrexone, oxytocin, ketamine, opioids |
| | | **Nerve Damage:** gabapentin, clonidine, topiramate, diazepam, carisoprodol, clonazepam, duloxetine, pregabalin |
| | | **Central/Electrical Agents:** amphetamine salts (Adderall®), methylphenidate (Ritalin®), phentermine, modafinil, tizanidine |
| **Non-Prescription Drugs** | **Non-Prescription Drugs** | **Non-Prescription Drugs** |
| curcumin/turmeric, serrapeptase, adrenal extract | gonadal extract (Orchex®), deer antler velvet, colostrum, pregnenolone, DHEA | palmitoylethanolamide (PEA), cannabinoid oils (CBD), kratom, corydalis, valerian |

# 47. PAIN FLARES

Every person with AA needs to be prepared for a pain flare. Don't kid yourself into thinking it won't happen. Most people with AA encounter an occasional, disabling flare. It's a little demoralizing, but flares occur without explanation. Don't blame yourself or the treatment that keeps you stable 90% of the time.

[79]

There are several options for flare treatment. We list some here as flare medication should be in your home ready to be used as soon as you know a flare is coming.

Here are some choices, but you may discover something better:
1. Ketorolac injection 30-60 mg for 2 days with or without methylprednisolone 20-30 mg
2. 6-Day methylprednisolone (Medrol® Dose Pak)
3. Suppository of hydromorphone 3 mg.
4. Suppositories of diazepam (Valium®) 5 to 10mg.
5. Patch of lidocaine, diclofenac or other.

# 48. SELF-HELP MEDICATION PROTOCOL

AA is a progressive, neuroinflammatory disease. <u>EVERY DAY</u> you delay treatment puts you at greater risk for increased pain, suffering, paralysis, bladder dysfunction, bed-bound state, and early demise. Too many people with AA are looking and waiting for a doctor to treat them. While waiting you must get started with treatment yourself.

Take at least <u>one</u> (two is usually better) of the non-prescription drugs listed in <u>each</u> component. These are available in health food stores or on the internet. Follow the dosage on the label except for pregnenolone and DHEA. The dosage for these hormones is listed here:

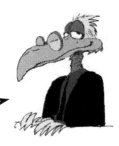

Dr. Beak says: Don't delay. Start today! The drugs listed don't need a doctor's prescription.

| SUPPRESSION OF NEUROINFLAMMATION | PROMOTION OF NEUROREGENERATION | CONTROL OF PAIN |
|---|---|---|
| Curcumin/Turmeric<br>Serrapeptase<br>Bovine Adrenal Extract | Pregnenolone and/or<br>DHEA<br>   *Start pregnenolone or DHEA at 50 mg a day and increase slowly as tolerated up to 200 to 400 mg a day.*<br>Colostrum<br>Collagen Preparations *(Gummies, Capsules, Liquid)*<br>Gonadal Extract (Orchex®)<br>Deer Antler Velvet | CBD Oil<br>Kratom<br>Palmitoylethanolamide (PEA)<br>Corydalis |

Start Today! The drugs listed here do not need a doctor's prescription. You can take non-prescription drugs with prescription drugs. Don't delay!

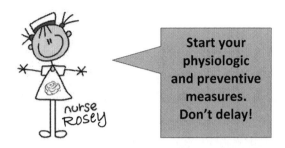

# 49. NEED FOR A COMPOUNDING PHARMACY

Compared to hypertension and asthma, AA is a "rare" disease. Proper treatment will, therefore, require some unusual medications. "Unusual" means a medication that isn't commercially available in most drug stores.

Listed here are compounded medications which are now regularly used by AA persons:

1. Ketorolac: 15, 30, or 60 mg – troche
2. Oxytocin: 40 or 80 units – troche or sublingual tablet
3. Ketamine: 25 or 50 mg per ml sublingual liquid
4. Nandrolone: 25 to 50 mg troche
5. Human Chorionic Gonadotropin (HCG): 250 to 500 units - troche, sublingual tablet, or injection
6. Low Dose Naltrexone (LDN): .5 to 2 mg capsule
7. Diazepam (Valium®) suppositories 5-10mg

Every person with AA should take this list to their local compound pharmacy and determine their cost and capability to make the above compounded medications.

# 50. I'M GETTING WORSE, WHAT DO I DO?

In our experience almost every person with AA who is progressively getting worse is only using symptomatic drugs for pain relief and not taking the drugs that suppress neuroinflammation or regenerate damaged nerves. Keep this key point always in mind. AA is a neuroinflammatory disease of the lumbar-sacral nerve roots and arachnoid covering of the spinal canal which may progressively destroy additional tissue. Worsening simply means you are neither suppressing neuroinflammation nor regrowing damaged nerve tissue.

Follow These Steps

1. Review the drugs that are in each of the 3 treatment components: (1) neuroinflammation suppression; (2) neuroregeneration; and (3) pain control. If you are not taking at least 1 drug in each component, you can expect to get worse.

2. Review the physiologic measures in this handout which involves spinal fluid flow, oxygen level, electricity retention, and tissue shrinkage prevention. Are you walking and doing other physiologic measures each day? Have your medical practitioner do a blood test for these hormones and replenish any that are low: cortisol, DHEA, estradiol, pregnenolone, progesterone, testosterone.

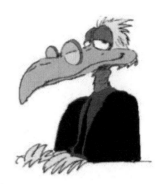

**Note:** Some people claim they can't take ketorolac or a "steroid" (i.e. methylprednisolone or dexamethasone). These can almost always be taken at a low dose as seldom as once a week and be effective.

3. We have found only 7 drugs to be consistently effective in controlling AA: ketorolac, methylprednisolone, dexamethasone, acetazolamide, low dose naltrexone, human chorionic gonadotropin (HCG), nandrolone. If you are not taking at least 2 of these 7, we believe you may get worse. Find out which ones your medical practitioner will prescribe.

4. If you feel your pain is worse, review the agents for pain control in this handbook. If you have constant pain, you may need a central electrical agent such as amphetamine salts (Adderal®). If you can only get a limited supply of opioids, take one or two of these non-prescription pain relievers: palmitoylethanolamide (PEA), cannabinoid oil (CBD), kratom, corydalis. Take them simultaneously with your opioid and/or between opioid dosages.

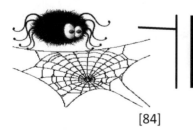

Happy Spider says:
If your doctor won't help, look for a new one!

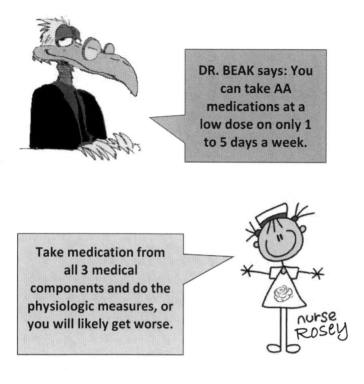

# 51. PSYCHOLOGICAL TREATMENT AND SUPPORT

AA is a frightening disease as it carries a high risk of severe disability, pain, misery, and a shortened life. It can also produce depression and loss of mental capacity.

Today there are psychologists who specialize in pain matters. They can often help you find comfort and peace. Mainly, they may be able to help you put together a game plan on how you are going to accomplish your therapeutic goals and simultaneously cope and maintain the other aspects of your life. Don't settle for any old therapist. Seek out only those that understand AA and constant, incurable pain.

[85]

## 52. SUPPORT GROUPS AND PARTNERS

Every person with AA needs to have a partner or buddy who has AA. It may take a while but find at least one other person with AA with whom you can share your goals, fears, and hopes. Today, thanks to computer technology, you can find social media group members who have AA. Your partner or buddy may be someone you find online. Our caution about groups and partners is negativism. Find people and groups who are positive about life and AA treatment potential.

## 53. YOUR FAMILY AND YOUR RELIGION

Too many people with AA feel ashamed and isolated. They even feel they are somehow to be blamed or even cursed by the devil. Get rid of these false beliefs. If you're lucky enough to have a loving spouse, share all. Next best is a family member you love and trust. People close to you need to know you have a serious disease of the spinal cord. This is as important as your physicians and medical help.

We highly recommend you have a clergyman with whom you can discuss your case. Whatever your religion and beliefs, please become better acquainted with your spiritual advisor. This handbook's goal is to give you the best guidance we can give. Be clearly advised. We have seen that deep religious and spiritual beliefs sometimes bring about healing, comfort, and well-being beyond our medical treatments and expectations.

# 54. WHEN AN ELECTRICAL STIMULATOR OR SPINAL CANAL INFUSION DEVICE ARE NEEDED

The physiologic measures and 3-component medical treatment described in this handbook have been developed over the past 10 years. Thanks to this research and development, fewer and fewer people with AA are ending up in the severe and catastrophic categories. People with AA who have had their disease over 5 years and who have not had the benefits of either physiologic measures or 3-component medical treatment may have so much nerve root adhesion, entrapment, damage, and scarring that pain cannot be relieved by the use of the medicinal agents described in this handbook. Another disabling factor in long-term, untreated people with AA is the additional pain caused by autoimmunity. In these situations, a trial with an implanted electrical stimulator and/or spinal canal (intrathecal) infusion device is warranted.

People with AA who possibly might need high dose opioid therapy may need to have it administered by injection, sublingual formulation, or by infusion directly into the spinal canal. A special implanted device is necessary to administer opioids directly into the spinal fluid. Those devices are often called "intrathecal pumps."

It is critical to understand that implanted electrical stimulators and high dose opioids are only symptomatic pain relievers that enhance physiologic functions, activities of daily living, and a meaningful life. They do not stop or slow the progression of AA. It is, therefore, critical that the medical components of neuroinflammation suppression and neuroregeneration be simultaneously administered with an implanted electrical stimulator and/or high dose opioid therapy given by injection, sublingual formulations, or intraspinal administration. The physiologic and preventive measures described in this handbook should also be continued.

## 55. EPIDURAL CORTICOSTEROID INJECTIONS AND SPINAL TAPS

Once a person has developed AA, an injection of any sort that goes into the epidural space or the spinal canal is not recommended except in lifesaving situations. The reason here is more intuitive than based on any scientific data. Here is our logic. AA is a neuroinflammatory disease of the nerve roots in the cauda equina and the arachnoid covering of the spinal canal. Since neuroinflammation is present, it seems logical that any chemical intrusion or trauma might aggravate or cause more neuroinflammation. It is also now known that there are micro-conduits between the epidural space and the interior of the spinal canal. This is how chemicals injected into the epidural space may enter the spinal fluid.

If a person who has AA wants to try an epidural corticosteroid injection, our recommendation is that the person, family, and physician be aware and acknowledge that there is an unknown risk as to whether AA may worsen with the procedure.

Spinal taps also carry a risk to the person with AA, since the needle must penetrate the arachnoid lining. In our opinion, they should only be done in the case of a life-threatening emergency in people with AA.

[88]

# 56. INFUSIONS OF LIDOCAINE, KETAMINE, AND VITAMIN C

As this handbook is being written, we are receiving more and more positive feedback on intravenous infusions of lidocaine, Vitamin C, and ketamine. They don't work for every person, but they are often providing about 1 to 3 months of comfort and reduced pain in many people with AA. The best news is that reports of side-effects are minimal. In other words, the benefits seem to outweigh the risks. Although the future may change our mind, we currently recommend these infusions to AA persons who are already on a 3-component medical program along with physiologic and preventive measures. Also, our research and education project are encouraging medical providers to provide intravenous infusions as positive ancillary measures people with AA.

# 57. GENETIC PREDISPOSING SUSCEPTIBILITY TO AA

There is now the belief among some medical practitioners and that some persons are susceptible to developing AA after an epidural injection, spinal tap, or trauma including surgery. Certainly, people with a genetic collagen disorder are susceptible and should consider avoiding any and all trauma in and around the spinal canal such as an epidural injection and surgery. People who have an autoimmune disorder such as psoriasis or systemic lupus erythematosus may also be susceptible. This is an area of research and persons with these conditions should be aware that they may have a genetic susceptibility to AA.

# 58. NO DOCTOR WILL HELP ME

Keep looking. Don't forget that almost every community has nurse practitioners (NP) and/or physician assistants (PA) who can prescribe. Oftentimes the NP's and PA's are more interested in assisting those with long-term illnesses, such as, AA than many MD's.

We are much better off today relative to physician access than we were 2 years ago. There is more and more awareness that AA is in every community and that it must be treated.

While looking for medical help, start the self-help medical protocol and physiologic measures provided in this handbook. It is intentionally designed with all non-prescription medications. It may even suffice for some mild cases. The self-help protocol may go a long way toward slowing or stopping the disease of AA until you can obtain more potent prescription drugs.

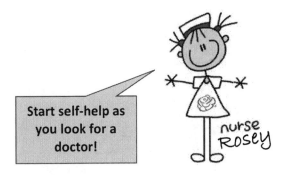

Start self-help as you look for a doctor!

nurse Rosey

When you go to a doctor, bring written materials about AA and documentation that you have AA. Tell him or her that you have most of the 4 cardinal symptoms: (1) pain that improves when reclining (2) bladder impairment; (3) feeling of water or bugs on your legs; and (4) burning feet. Know ahead of time what your insurance will pay for and where you can obtain supplies. Know which compounding pharmacy can make any supplies that are not carried by a standard pharmacy. Ask other people with AA about which doctor to seek out. Be prepared to travel some distance to a knowledgeable doctor. Be prepared to tell a medical practitioner which drugs you want to try and that you know the risks and benefit of treatment.

# 59. THE 21 DAY RULE

Each person with AA must develop their own medication program with the help of their medical provider. We strongly advise a 3-component medication approach as described in this handbook. We present several agents in each component that we believe to be effective in some people with AA. You will have to try different medications to build an effective program. Which ones you end up with depend on multiple factors including allergy, side-effects, and cost.

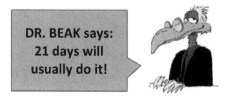

DR. BEAK says:
21 days will
usually do it!

As you try different medications and dosages, we recommend the 21-day rule. Take any new medication for 21 days. If you can't tell an improvement in pain control, energy, motivation, comfort, or mental ability, stop the medication. Don't keep taking a medication that you are unsure about, because one medication may render another one to be ineffective.

When you stop a medication, sometimes you feel worse and realize the medication was helping. In this case just restart the medication.

# 60. HOW TO DEAL WITH OPIOID RESTRICTIONS

Opioid prescribing restrictions and poor availability of opioids is now standard. Each state is slightly different. There is a maximal amount of daily opioid recommended by the United States Centers for Disease Control and Prevention (CDC). They recommend a daily 90 mg limit called a morphine milligram equivalence (MME). Physicians can prescribe higher levels if they justify the need. However, physicians must limit their opioid prescribing to comply with their state and local restrictions. Some physicians are also restricted by their malpractice carrier or employer. The federal government and state pharmacy boards are progressively limiting supplies in pharmacies. Some veteran's hospitals have essentially banned opioids.

From a practical standpoint, we recommend that every person with AA pick a strategy to find relief with zero or limited amounts of opioids. A federal 90 mg morphine equivalence table is given here to provide a rough idea as to the maximal amount of daily opioid that can be prescribed in most locations.

| | MAXIMAL DAILY OPIOID DOSAGES ALLOWED |
|---|---|
| **Approx. Oral Doses a Day** | **OPIOID (Oral or Patch)** |
| 8-9 | Morphine – 10 mg |
| 3-4 | Methadone – 10 mg |
| 8-9 | Hydrocodone/APAP – 10/325 mg (Vicodin®, Norco®) |
| 3 | Morphine – 30 mg |
| 6 | Oxycodone/APAP – 10/325 mg (Percocet®) |
| 5 | Hydromorphone – 4 mg (Dilaudid®) |
| 2-3 | Hydromorphone – 8 mg (Dilaudid®) |
| 6 | Oxycodone Plain – 10 mg |
| 2-3 | Oxycodone Plain – 20 mg |
| 2 | Oxycodone Plain – 30 mg |
| 16-20 | Codeine 30 mg |
| 8-10 | Codeine 60 mg |
| 16-18 | Tramadol 50 mg |
| 8-9 | Tramadol 100 mg |
| 1 | Fentanyl Patch – 25 mcg per hour |
| 1 | Fentanyl Patch – 50 mcg per hour is 120 mg of morphine equivalence |
| | **OPIOID INJECTIONS** |
| 2-4 | Hydromorphone 50 mg/ml, .05 to .1 ml (2.5 to 5 mg) |
| 3-4 | Fentanyl 1000 mcg/ml, 0.1 ml (100 mcg) sub cu per injection |
| 8-9 | Morphine 10 mg per injection |
| 3-4 | Meperidine (Demerol®) 50-100 mg per injection |
| • | This table is based on recommendations of the Federal Centers for Medicare and Medicaid. |
| • | If a person wishes, they can take 2 opioids, each at half the maximal number a day which is listed above. |

# 61. THREE STRATEGIES TO DEAL WITH OPIOID RESTRICTION

Here are 3 strategies to deal with the limited availability of opioids. If you are unable to get the amounts of opioids you would like, review these 3 strategies and select one.

## Strategy No. 1 – Comprehensive, Symptomatic Pain Relief

Take one or more pain reliever from each of the 6 categories listed here. Many people on prescription opioids prescribed by their doctor don't use a comprehensive pain control program and rely solely on opioids.

1. Opioid – hydrocodone, oxycodone, morphine, hydromorphone, tapentadol
2. Non-opioid Pain Relievers – ketamine, oxytocin, corydalis, CBD oil, PEA, kratom, valerian
3. Neuropathic (injured nerve) – gabapentin, topiramate, carisoprodol, diazepam
4. Electrical/Central/Descending – amphetamine, methylphenidate, phentermine, modafinil, tizanidine
5. Bedtime Aid/Pain Reliever – clonidine, gabapentin
6. Topical/Skin – Lidocaine patch or gel

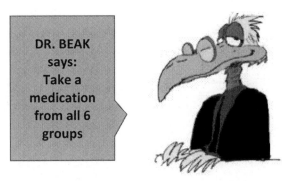

**DR. BEAK says: Take a medication from all 6 groups**

[94]

## Strategy No. 2 – Potentiate or "Boost" Opioid Effectiveness for Maximal Pain Relief

Take agents that boost opioid power. Take your opioid on a regular, same time each day basis, such as every 4 to 6 hours. Take a potentiator or booster simultaneously with your opioid and between opioid dosages. Example: Take hydrocodone with corydalis. One or two hours later, take another dose of corydalis.

Potentiator or Boosting Agents: corydalis, CBD products, kratom, palmitoylethanolamide (PEA), ketamine, oxytocin

## Strategy No. 3 – Treat Underlying Cause of Pain (AA)

We have found that the most effective way to reduce opioid dosage is to vigorously treat AA with a 3-component medication program plus physiologic measures.

## Anti-Neuroinflammatory Agents - Examples

1. Ketorolac – 2 to 3 days a week
2. Methylprednisolone or dexamethasone – 3 days a week
3. Acetazolamide – 5 days a week

> **DR. BEAK says: The best strategy to lower opioid dosage is vigorous treatment of the disease that is causing pain.**

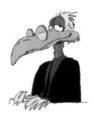

## Neuroregenerative Agents - Examples

1. Pregnenolone and/or DHEA 200 to 300 mg 2-3 times a week
2. Nandrolone troche– 25 mg on 3 to 5 days a week
3. Human Chorionic Gonadotropin (HCG) – 500 units on 3 days a week

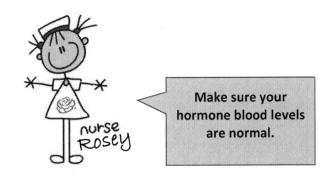

**For all 3 strategies, replenish any of these hormones that are deficient in the blood: pregnenolone, DHEA, testosterone.**

SPECIAL NOTE: Parts of all 3 strategies may be more effective than one alone.

# 62. DEALING WITH THE FEAR OF HORMONES

The American public and the average doctor has become unduly afraid of hormones. This has been brought about by incessant, negative propaganda about their possible complications. Vested financial interests have grossly overblown the cases of estrogen or testosterone administration that caused breast, uterine, or testicular cancer. The term "steroid" has become a synonymous term with cortisone when it is the chemical structure that is the basis of almost all hormones, that are made by the body.

Those of us who constantly work with hormones know precisely why vested pharmacologic interests have done their best to keep people and practitioners away from hormones. They simply are very effective in both prevention and treatment of many medical conditions. We consider the use of some hormones, or their synthetic derivatives, to be essential in the treatment of AA.

Be advised. The frightening reports about cancer, bone degeneration (osteoporosis), and impotence with hormones were all based on persons who took high dosages of a hormone on a regular, daily basis. No wonder complications occurred. Check it out. Hormones for AA including corticoids are taken in low or modest dosages on only some days each week or month. Hormone complications are best avoided by using them on a low dosage intermittent basis.

We describe here some of the hormones you will need, in our experience, to slow or stop progression of your disease and find some relief and recovery. First, some cortisone derivatives are the most potent suppressors of neuroinflammation. The most effective are methylprednisolone (Medrol®) and dexamethasone (Decadron®). People with AA can take a low oral dosage of either hormone on 2 or 3 days a week. Some people take an injection of methylprednisolone 1 to 4 times a month (e.g. weekly). A Medrol® six-day dosage package is a good flare or emergency treatment.

A recent research discovery has found that the spinal cord and brain make some specific hormones which are called neurosteroids. Their function is to protect nerve cells from inflammation and regrow damaged cells (neuroregeneration). These hormones include pregnenolone, DHEA, progesterone, and estradiol. Although these neurosteroids are in an early stage of clinical use, we find them to be useful for people with AA. We recommend a blood test to see if any are depleted and need replenishment. Each can be given a 21-day trial.

There are now some hormone products that people with AA can obtain without a prescription. In case you can't find a doctor, who will prescribe hormones, you should obtain one or more of the non-prescription hormonal agents. These include adrenal and gonadal extracts, colostrum, and deer antler velvet. Neither pregnenolone nor DHEA require a prescription. The dosage is 200 to 300 mg taken at one time on 3 to 5 days a week.

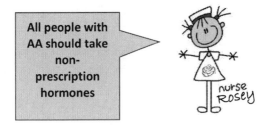

[98]

# 63. HUMAN CHORIONIC GONADOTROPIN (HCG) AND NANDROLONE

These 2 hormonal agents are proving to be essential for some people with AA. HCG is the hormone whose natural function is to grow brain, spinal cord, skin, nails, and hair "ectoderm" tissue in the embryo. In the adult, its function is to maintain hormone levels of thyroid, progesterone, estradiol, and testosterone and regrow any damaged nerve tissue. Studies in laboratory animals show it can regenerate spinal cord tissue. Unfortunately, HCG has some prohibitive expense and availability for people with AA. Except for persons in the mild category, we recommend it as an injection, sublingual solution, or troche. Dosage is 250 to 500 units taken 2 to 5 times a week. We have observed some remarkable results including the elimination of paralysis and the reduction of pain great enough that opioids were no longer needed. Once people with AA have stabilized on some anti-neuroinflammation and pain control medication, we recommend a 3-month trial of HCG. Side-effects are seldom but may include acne and hair loss. If this occurs the dosage should be lowered. HCG can be stopped for a period and alternated with another hormone. We are aware of people with AA who have taken HCG for over 5 years and continue to recover. All people with AA are highly encouraged to locate a supplier and work with family, insurance carrier, or other party to finance a 3-month trial.

Nandrolone is a synthetic testosterone derivative approved by the US Food and Drug Administration (FDA) for regeneration of tissue in wasting states caused by a severe disease. AA qualifies. It will regenerate nerve, muscle, and other soft (non-bone) tissue. Although available as an expensive injectable compound, it can be made into a relatively inexpensive troche by compounding pharmacies. The starting troche dosage is 25 mg given on 3 to 5 days a week. Nandrolone has pain-relief properties.

We consider nandrolone almost essential for persons with the dual disease problem of a genetic collagen disorder (Ehlers-Danlos/Marfan types) and AA. All people with AA except those in the mild category should have, in our opinion, a 21-day trail of nandrolone. It works much faster than HCG, so persons usually feel a benefit within the first week.

HCG and nandrolone can be taken together. We have used both hormones in cases of AA with multiple spinal cord complications like Chiari herniations, syringomyelia, and Tarlov cysts. These two hormones can also be alternated. For example, one month of nandrolone and then rotate to HCG.

People with AA must realize that the use of these hormones is considered "revolutionary" in the minds of most physicians. They represent a departure from mainstream medical practice. Our answer is, simple. AA is a progressive, devastating disease unless treated. Genetic collagen disorders progressively dissolve collagen and render tissue painful and dysfunctional. As this handbook is being written (2019) we are becoming increasingly more adamant that these two hormones should become a "backbone" of treatment for the dual disease problem of AA and the genetic collagen disorders such as EDS. The benefit of the 2 hormones far outweigh the risks of AA and GCD.

# 64. MY MEDICATION PROGRAM HAS QUIT WORKING

When your medication program suddenly stops working, it is usually due to a lack of neuroinflammation control. Always remember that AA is a neuroinflammatory disease of the cauda equina nerve roots and the arachnoid covering of the spinal canal.

In our experience people with AA who complain of sudden lack of effectiveness of their medical protocol are usually not taking ketorolac and methylprednisolone (Medrol®) or its close relative, dexamethasone. Due to our clinical experience, we believe that at least a single dosage of ketorolac and methylprednisolone are necessary every 7 to 10 days unless the person with AA is in the "mild" category. Even then, occasional dosages of ketorolac and methylprednisolone are well-advised. These 2 drugs have emerged to be the backbone of AA treatment. Always keep in mind that neuroinflammation may be silently clumping and destroying your nerve roots. Consequently, you may suddenly, without warning, take a "turn for the worse."

Another reason your medication program may stop working is the development of a hormone deficiency of pregnenolone, progesterone, estradiol, or testosterone. A blood test is a wise move to determine if you have a deficiency. If so, replenishment of one or more hormones is necessary, as adequate hormone levels are necessary to make inflammatory and pain control drugs maximally effective.

Naturally, you will want to review the 3-medication components and physiologic measures presented in this handbook. Perhaps you need to change some drugs. Make sure you are taking agents from all 3-components and doing physiologic measures each day.

# 65. I CAN'T GET A DIAGNOSIS

Unfortunately, there is far too much reliance on the MRI to make the diagnosis of AA. A diagnosis of AA is rather clear cut. There is usually an initiating disease or event such as an accident or genetic disease. There are major symptoms: (1) pain decreases on reclining; (2) feeling of water or bugs on the legs; (3) urinary difficulty; and (4) burning ankles or feet. Physical exam usually shows some neurologic deficit in the legs or feet. The MRI confirms what the history and physical indicate.

Although it is changing, some communities and physicians still don't want to accept AA as a diagnosis or disease. They still remember the days of malpractice claims and blame over AA. They still believe that AA is only caused by physician error which today is rarely the case. Some radiologists just haven't seen it often enough to diagnose it. Another problem is that some MRI's don't show classic nerve root clumping and adhesions. This problem may be technical. An MRI is a series of photographs, and a small area of AA can be missed.

Please heed this advice. If you are sure that you have AA or it was diagnosed by physicians other than your primary doctors, let your doctors know this. If your doctors deny you have AA, simply ask them "What do I have?" and "What is the treatment you recommend?" We are aware that physicians in communities everywhere are beginning to diagnose and treat AA. Too many people now have AA to keep sweeping the diagnosis under the rug. Keep looking for a knowledgeable and willing doctor. They are "cropping up."

# 66. WHY CAN'T I GET BETTER?

There are usually one or two reasons why you may not get better. One is that you have had AA for a long time before any known treatment was available, and you simply have severe nerve damage that won't resolve or repair. The problem is that AA is a neuroinflammatory disease of the cauda equina nerve roots and arachnoid covering. Unfortunately, neuroinflammation can destroy nerve tissue to the point of scarring and permanent non-function. Pain relief and retention of some neurologic function may be the best you can do, but we highly recommend you attempt to get better, no matter how much damage or neurologic impairment you have.

Most people with AA don't get better because they don't have a good: 2 strategy treatment: (1) specific physiologic measures; and (2) 3-component medical program. To get better a person with AA must clearly understand the difference between "symptomatic" or "comfort" measures and "curative" or "improvement" measures.

<u>Here Are Some Examples of Curative or Improvement Measures and Drugs:</u>

<u>Physiologic Measures</u>
- ✓ Walking
- ✓ Water Soaking
- ✓ Stretching

<u>Improvement Medications</u>
- ✓ Ketorolac
- ✓ Methylprednisolone
- ✓ Human chorionic gonadotropin (HCG)
- ✓ Nandrolone

Many people with AA make this mistake. They get to feeling better with their new treatment, so they are satisfied. Don't do this as our culprit, neuroinflammation, may be lurking and doing silent damage. Push yourself to do more physiologic measures. For example, walk a little farther or stretch a little more. Keep up a vigorous hormone therapy program as these are the body's natural agents that suppress neuroinflammation and stimulate regrowth of damaged nerves.

## 67. AA TREATMENT IS PROTOCOL - NOT EVIDENCE-BASED

There is a great "fight" and controversy in today's medical practice. Some parties demand that any treatment, including drugs and other measures, be "evidence-based". The meaning here is that there must be double-blind, random, controlled studies or some other statistical parameter showing "evidence" before a treatment should be used. Naturally, the parties pushing for "evidence" are those paying the bills. They don't want to pay for anything that is not "evidence-based." In other words, "one size fits all", and there should be no payment or financing for any other treatment. Unfortunately, the cost and effort to do these types of studies is so prohibitive that only a small percentage of drugs and medical therapies can ever be tested under statistical control.

"Evidence -based" is not, however, the way medicine has always been practiced. Certainly, there will be more "evidence" in the future, but traditional medical practice will, for the foreseeable future, continue

[104]

to be protocol-based. Be clearly advised; another name for protocol is "old-fashioned common-sense medicine." All it means is that we have a basket of therapies. The medical provider is to pick one or two. Try them. If they work – terrific! If they don't, try another one. The idea is to take several measures, and through trial and error come up with a satisfactory treatment plan. AA is a complex neuroinflammatory disease of multiple causes and symptoms. No two persons will end up with precisely the same treatment program. Just like people with cardiac, pulmonary, or diabetic disorders, one size won't fit all. Remember this. If someone tells you that you need "evidence-based" treatment, stay with the drugs and therapies that you and your practitioner know work. Your comfort and well-being are the "best evidence."

# 68. RISK VS BENEFIT AND INFORMED CONSENT

You cannot find any relief or recovery with AA unless you are willing to take some risks. All the medications, including those that are non-prescription, have risks better known as side-effects and complications. Even the physiologic measures have risks. For example, you might overstretch or walk too far and tear apart an adhesion.

Here is the basic fact. All the best treatment agents identified to date for AA have risks. The best drugs and their best-known complications or side- effects are listed here:

1. Ketorolac – kidney damage
2. Methylprednisolone and Dexamethasone – osteoporosis, weight gain, hyperglycemia
3. Acetazolamide – dizziness, nausea, dysphoria (opposite of euphoria)
4. Human Chorionic Gonadotropin – acne, hair loss

5. Pregnenolone – acne, hair loss
6. Nandrolone – acne, hair loss
7. Naltrexone – increase in pain, dysphoria (opposite of euphoria)

Simply put, we don't believe you can find much long-term relief, much less recovery, unless you are taking at least a couple of the drugs listed above. You must accept their risks to get their benefit. AA is a progressive neuroinflammatory disease of cauda equina nerve roots. Unless controlled, it has serious sequelae with an autoimmune component and shortened life span. There is no more miserable disease or one that ruins a quality of life more drastically. What's important is that you inform your medical providers that you know the risks and are willing to accept them. This is known as "informed consent."

The best way, and it is our firm recommendation, to prevent complications is to take AA drugs on only 3 to 5 days a week or even monthly. Complications occur most often with daily use of a drug.

Ketorolac is a special case, and we make special note of it here as it is the most consistent drug for treatment of the neuroinflammation of AA. For over 2 decades it is known and labeled by the US Food and Drug Administration (FDA) that it cannot be taken for over five days in a row. We firmly agree. Some ill-informed persons in the medical field, especially some pharmacists, believe this means 5 days in a lifetime. This is not the case. We recommend that the maximal dosage be 3 days a week and that days must be skipped between dosages. If one is over 70 years old, we recommend that a kidney blood test for damage be done at least every 3 to 6 months.

[106]

We normally like to see the corticosteroids methylprednisolone and dexamethasone, only be taken on 2 to 3 days a week in a low, oral dosage. Some people with AA, however, find they can't function and experience unbearable pain without a higher dosage taken almost daily. There are obviously greater risks with higher dosages taken more frequently. Simply put, you may have to take more risk. Many people with AA and their physicians are learning that a periodic (e.g. 7-10 days interval) injection of about 10 to 20 milligrams of methylprednisolone may be more effective than oral dosages and have less risk.

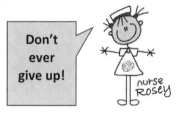

The take home message is this. AA, like cancer, is a devastating disease, and the drugs that treat it have risks that a person must accept to get their benefits and improve.

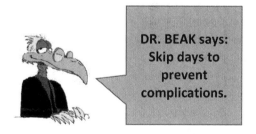

# 69. SUMMARY

The treatment strategy outlined in this handbook is two-fold: (1) medication and (2) physiologic and preventive measures. Medication administration has 3-components: (1) suppression of neuroinflammation; (2) regrowth of damaged nerves (neuroregeneration); and (3) pain control.  The first goal of treatment is to "not get worse!"

Once a person is on a 3-componant medical protocol with accompanying physiologic and preventative measures, we highly recommend electromagnetic therapy, intravenous infusions, and other potential experimental measures such as stem cells. There are four categories of AA severity; mild, moderate, severe, and catastrophic. Some people with AA who are in the severe or catastrophic categories will require the implantation of an electric stimulator or opioid infusion pump for symptomatic pain relief.

Medical providers are just starting to understand and treat AA.  Some uninformed providers still deny and reject it as a disease, but they will change in the future because AA is increasing in the population.  In the meantime, every person with AA and their family needs to start self-help treatment with the help of the measures and suggestions in this handbook.

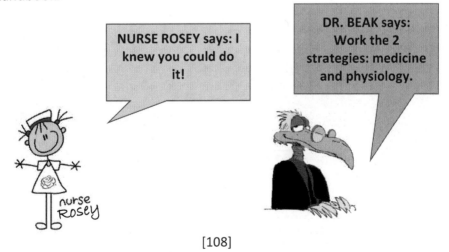

**NURSE ROSEY says: I knew you could do it!**

**DR. BEAK says: Work the 2 strategies: medicine and physiology.**

nurse Rosey

[108]

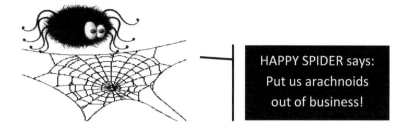

HAPPY SPIDER says:
Put us arachnoids
out of business!

DISCLAIMER: No content in this handbook can be considered a medical order or advice. All materials and recommendations of the authors are based on experience and research. No guarantees or assurances can be derived from this handbook. All medical advice must come from a licensed medical practitioner who has examined and evaluated a person who is their patient.

PROHIBITION: No portion of this handbook may be copied or published anywhere, including internet and social media without the written permission of the authors.

# THE FOE CHART of PHYSIOLOGIC MEASURES

| | |
|---|---|
| F- | Flow of Spinal Fluid - "Power Walking" |
| O- | Oxygen Intake- "Deep Breathing" |
| E- | Electricity Elimination- "Water Soak" |
| S- | Seepage and Shrinkage- "Stretch and Extend Arms and Legs" |

Neuroinflammation and adhesions are our **FOES**

**THINK FOES**

nurse Rosey

Simple measures will send me packing

# REFERENCES

HISTORY

1. Thomas J. Arachnitis and Arachnoiditis. *Comprehensive Medical Dictionary.* Philadelphia, J.B. Lippincott & Co. 1873; p57.
2. Aldrete JA. History and evaluation of arachnoiditis: the evidence revealed. Insurgentes Centro 51-A. Col San Rafael, Mexico 2010; p3-14.
3. Horsley VAH. Chronic spinal meningitis: its differential diagnosis and surgical treatment. Br J Med 1909; 1:513-517.
4. Charcot JM, Joffrey A. Deax cas d'atrophic musculaire progressive avec lesions de a substance gris et des faisceaux anterolateraux de la moelle spinaire. Arch de Physiologic 1869; 2:354-358.
5. Addison T. The constitutional and local effects of disease of the supra-renal capsules. London: Samuel Highley;1855.
6. Elliott J. Of the cure of sciatica in a complete collection of the medical and philosophical works of John Fothergill. Pater-Nofter-Row, London;1781: p355-363.
7. Meningitis, Cerebral, Spinal, and Tubercular in Merck's 1899 Manual of the Materia Medica: A Ready Reference Pocket Book for the Practicing Physician. Merck & Co. New York, 1899; p146.
8. Harvey SC. Meningeal adhesions and their significance. Interstate Post Grad Med, North America Prac 1926;2:27-31.

DIAGNOSIS

9. Quiles M, Marchiselo PJ, Tsairis P. Lumbar adhesive arachnoiditis: etiologic and pathologic aspects. Spine 1978; 3:45-50.
10. Burton C. Lumbosacral arachnoiditis. Spine 1978; 3:24-30.
11. Jackson A, Isherwood I. Does degenerative disease of the lumbar spine cause arachnoiditis? A magnetic resonance study and review of the literature. Brit J Radiology 1994; 67:840-847.
12. Aldrete JA. Suspecting and diagnosing arachnoiditis. Pract Pain Mgt 2006;16(5):74-87.
13. Tennant F. Arachnoiditis: clinical description. Pract Pain Mgt 2016;14(7):63-69.
14. Tennant F. Erythrocyte sedimentation rate and C-reactive protein: old but useful biomarkers for pain treatment. Pract Pain Mgt. 2013;13(2):61-65.
15. Tennant F. Arachnoiditis: diagnosis and treatment. *Pract Pain Mgt* 2016; 16(5):74-87.
16. Tennant FS. Hormone abnormalities in severe chronic pain persons who fail standard treatment. Postgrad Med 2015;127(1):1-4.

## TREATMENT

17. O'Callgan JP, SriranT, Miller DB. Defining "neuroinflammation". Ann NY Acad Sci 2008; 1139:318-330.
18. Tsuda M. Microglia in the spinal cord and neuropathic pain. J Diabetes Investig 2016;7(1):17-26.
19. Loggia MI, Chunde DB, Oluwaseum A, et al. Evidence for brain glial activation in chronic pain persons. Brain 2015; 138:604-615.
20. Mika J. Modulation of microglia can attenuate neuropathic pain symptoms and enhance morphine effectiveness. Pharmacol Rep 2008; 60:297-300.
21. Bilello J, Tennant F. Patterns of chronic inflammation in extensively treated persons with arachnoiditis and chronic intractable pain. Postgrad Med 2016;92(17):1-5.
22. Compagnone NA, Mellon SH. Neurosteroids: biosynthesis and function of these novel neuromodulators. Front Neuroendocrinol 2000; 21:1-56.
23. Jones KJ. Gonadal steroids and neuronal regeneration: a therapeutic role. Adv Neurol 1993; 59:227-240.
24. Joels M, DeKloet E. Control of neuronal excitability by corticosteroid hormones. Trends Neurosci 1992; 15:25-30.
25. Guth L, Zhang Z, Roberts E. Key role for pregnenolone in combination therapy that promotes recovery after spinal cord injury. Proc Natl Acad Sci 1994; 91:12308-12312.
26. Kilts JD, Tupler LA, Keefe FJ, et al. Neurosteroids and self-reported pain in veterans who served in the military after September 11,2001. Pain Med 2010; 10:1469-1476.
27. He J, Evans CO, Hoffman SW, et al. Progesterone and allopregnanolone reduce inflammatory cytokines after traumatic brain injury. Exp Neuro 2004; 189:404-412.
28. Patil AA. The effect of human chorionic gonadotropin (HCG) on restoration of the spinal cord: A preliminary report. Int Surg 1990;75(1):54-57.
29. Inyang K, Szabo-Pardi T, Price T. Treatment of chronic pain: long-term effects of metformin on chronic neuropathic pain and microglial activation. Poster presented at Annual Meeting of the American Pain Society, May 11-14, 2016; Austin, TX Poster 309.
30. Aldrete JA. Epidural injections of indomethacin for post-laminectomy syndrome: a preliminary report. Anesth Anal 2003;96(2):463-468.

31. Nakano M, Matsui H, Miaki K, et al. Post-laminectomy adhesion of the cauda equina: inhibitory effects of anti-inflammatory drugs on cauda equina adhesion in rats. Spine 1998;23(3):298-304.
32. Tawfik VL, Nutile-McMenemy N, Lacroix-Fralish MI, et al. Efficacy of propentofylline, a glial modulating agent, on existing mechanical allodynia following peripheral nerve injury. Brain Behav Immun 2007; 21:238-246.
33. Tikka TM, Kaistinaha JE. Minocycline provides neuroprotection against n-methyl-d-asparate neurotoxicity by inhibiting microglia. J Immunol 66:7527=7533.
34. Mika J. Modulation of microglia can attenuate neuropathic pain symptoms and enhance morphine effectiveness. Pharmacol Rep 2008; 60:297-300.
35. Radhakrishnan R, Sluka KA. Acetazolamide, a carbonic anhydrase inhibitor, reverses inflammation-induced thermal hyperalgesia in rats. J Pharmacol Exp Ther 2005; 313:921-927.
36. Harvey JW, Otterson M, Yun H, et al. Acetazolamide reduces referred postoperative pain after laparoscopic surgery with carbon dioxide insufflation. Anesthesiology 2003; 99:924-928.)
37. Liu J, Feng X, Yu M, et al. Pentoxifylline attenuates the development of hyperalgesia in a rat model of neuropathic pain. Neurosci Lett 2007; 412:268-272.
38. Vale ML, Benevides VM, Sachs D, et al. Antihyperalgesic effect of pentoxifylline on experimental inflammatory pain. Br J Pharmacol 2004; 143:833-844.
39. Asiedu M, Ossipov MHG, Kaila K, et al. Acetazolamide and midazolam act synergistically to inhibit neuropathic pain. Pain 2010;148(2):302-308.
40. Pi R, Wenning L, Nelson TK, et al. Minocycline prevents glutamate-induced apoptosis of cerebellar granule neurons by differential regulation of p38 and akt pathways. J Neurochem 2004; 91:1219-1230.
41. Tikka T, Usenius T, Tenhunon M, et al. Tetracycline derivatives and ceftriaxone, a cephalospaorin antibiotic, protect neurons against apoptosis induced by ionizing radiation. J Neurochem 2001; 78:1409-1414.
42. Pabreja K, Dua K, Sharma S, et al. Minocycline attenuates the development of diabetic neuropathic pain: possible anti-inflammatory and antioxidant mechanism. Eur J Pharmacol 2011;661(1-3):15-21.
43. Liu J, Li W, Zhu J, et al. The effect of pentoxifylline on existing hypersensitivity in a rat model of neuropathy. Anaesth Analog 2008; 106:650-653.
44. Singh R, Sen I, Wig J, et al. An acetazolamide based multimodal analgesic approach versus conventional pain management in persons undergoing laparoscopic living donor. Indian J Anaesth 2009;53(4):434-441.
45. George C, Lefain JL, Delonion S. Case report: resolution of symptomatic epidural fibrosis following treatment with combined pentoxifylline-tocopherol. Br J Radiol 2004; 77:885-887.

46. Delanian S, Porcher R, Balla-Mekias S, et al. Randomized placebo-controlled trial of combined pentoxifylline and tocopherol for regression of superficial radiation-induced fibrosis. J Clin Oncol 2003; 21:2545-2550.
47. Lefaix JL, Delanizan S, Vozenin MC, et al. Striking regression of subcutaneous fibrosis induced by high doses of gamma rays using a combination of pentoxifylline and alpha tocopherol: an experimental study. Int J Radiat Oncol Biol Phys 1999; 43:839-847.
48. Compagnone NA, Mellon SH. Neurosteroids: biosynthesis and function of these novel neuromodulators. Front Neuroendocrinol 2000; 21:1-56
49. Mensah-Nyagan A.G., Meyer L., Schaeffer V., et al. Evidence for a key role of steroids in the modulation of pain. Psychoneuroendocrinology, Volume 34, Issue SUPPL. 1, 2009, S169-S177.
50. Reddy DS. Neurosteroids: endogenous role in the human brain and therapeutic potentials. Prog Brain Res 2010; 186:13-137.
51. Dawson-Basoa M, Gintzler AR. Estrogen and progesterone activate spinal kappa-opiate receptor analgesic mechanisms. Pain 1996;64: 608-615.
52. Ceccon M, Runbaugh G, Vincini S. Distinct effect of pregnenolone sulfate on NMDA receptor subtypes. Neuropharm 2001; 40:491-500.
53. Frye CA, Duncan JE. Progesterone metabolites, effective at the GABA(A) receptor complex, attenuate pain sensitivity in rats. Brain Res 1994; 643:194-23.
54. Garcia-Estrada J, Luquin S, Fernandez AM, et al. Dehydroepiandrosterone, pregnenolone, and sex steroids down-regulate reactive astroglia in the male rat brain after a penetrating brain injury. Intern J Develop Neuro 1999;17(2):145-151.
55. Evrard HC, Balthazart J. Rapid regulation of pain by estrogens synthesized in spinal dorsal horn neurons. J Neurosci 2004; 24:7225-7229.
56. Webster KM, Wright DK, Sun M, et al. Progesterone treatment reduces neuroinflammation, oxidative stress and brain damage and improves long-term outcomes in a rat model of repeated mild traumatic brain injury. J Neuroinflammation 2015 Dec 18;12-238.
57. Chang DM, Chu SJ, Chen HC, et al. Dehydroepiandrosterone suppresses interleukin 10 synthesis in women with systemic lupus erythematosus. Ann Rheum Dis 2004; 63:1623-1620.
58. McEwen BS, de Kloet ER, Rostene W. Adrenal steroid receptors and action in the central nervous system. Physio Rev 1986; 66:1121-1188.

59. Joels M, DeKloet E. Control of neuronal excitability by corticosteroid hormones. Trends Neurosci 1992; 15:25-30.
60. Bohn MC, O'Banion NK, Young DA, et al. In vitro studies of glucocorticoid effects on neurons and astrocytes. Amer NY Acad Sci 1994; 746:243-258.
61. Roglio I, Bianchi R, Gotti S, et al. Neuroprotective effects of dehydroprogesterone and progesterone in an experimental model of nerve crush injury. Neurosci 2008 Aug 26;155(3):673-685.
62. Djeball M, Guo Q, Pertus EH, et al. The neurosteroids progesterone and allopregnanolone reduce cell death, gliosis, and functional deficits after traumatic brain injury in rats. J Neurotrauma 2005; 22:106-118.
63. Morlin R, Young J, Corpechot C, et al. Neurosteroids: pregnenolone in human sciatic nerves. Proc Natl Acad Sci 1992; 98:6790-793.
64. Akwa Y, Young J, Kabbadj K, et al. Neurosteroids: biosynthesis, metabolism and function of pregnenolone and dehydroepiandrosterone in the brain. J Steroid Biochem Molec Biol 1991:40(1-3):71-81.
65. Jones KJ. Gonadal steroids and neuronal regeneration: a therapeutic role. Adv Neurol 1993; 59:227-240.
66. Fednekar J and Mulgacnker V. Role of testosterone on pain threshold in rats. Indian J Physci Pharmacol 1995; 39:423-24.
67. Hau M, Dominguez OA, Evrard HC. Testosterone reduces responsiveness to nociceptive stimuli in a wild bird. Horm Behav 2004; 46:165-170.
68. Aloisi AM, Ceccarelli I, Fiorenzani P, et al. Testosterone affects pain-related responses differently in male and female rats. Neurosci Lett. 2004; 361:262-264.
69. Matura S, Okashi M, Chen HC, et al. Physiochemical and Immunological Characterization of an HCG-Like Substance from human pituitary glands. Nature 1980; 286: 740-741.
70. Lei ZM, Rao CV. Neural actions of luteinizing hormone and human chorionic gonadotropin. Seminar Reprod Med 2001; 19:103-109.
71. Lei ZM, Rao CV, Kornyei JL, et al. Novel expression of human chorionic gonadotropin/luteinizing hormone receptor gene in brain. Endocrin 1993; 132:2262-2270.
72. Tennant F. Human chorionic gonadotropin in pain treatment. Prac Pain Mgt 2009; 9:44-46.
73. Vielkind U, Walencewicz A, Levine JM, et al. Type II glucocorticoid receptors are expressed in oligodendrocytes and astrocytes. J Neurosci Res 1990;27(3):360-323.
74. Kiefer r, Kreutzberg GW. Effects of dexamethasone on microglial activation in vitro: selective downregulation of major histocompatibility complex class II expression in regenerating facial nucleus. J Neuroimmunol 1991;34(2-3):99-108.
75. Chao CC, Hu S, Close K, et al. Cytokine release from microglia: differential inhibition by pentoxifylline and dexamethasone. J Infect Dis 1992;166(4):842-853.

76. Tanaka J, Fujita H, Mostsudo S, et al. Glucocorticoid and mineral corticoid receptors in microglial cells: the two receptors mediate differentiation effects of corticosteroids. Glia 1997; 20:23-37.
77. Rash JA, Aguirre-Camancho A, Campbell TS. Oxytocin and pain: a systemic review and synthesis of findings. Clin J Pain 2014;30(5):453-462.
78. Paloyells Y, Krahe C, Mahazos S, et al. The analgesic effect of oxytocin in humans: a double-blind placebo controlled cross-over study using easer-evoked potentials. J Neuroendocrinol 2016;28(4):10,111.
79. Tennant F, Pedersen C. Sublingual oxytocin and ketamine for pain relief. Poster Presented at PainWeek. September 5-9, 2017. Las Vegas, Nevada.
80. Gold J, High HA, Li Y, et al. Safety and efficacy of nandrolone decanoate for treatment of wasting in persons with HIV infection. AIDS 1996 Jun;10(7):745-52.
81. Sattler FR, Jaque SV, Schroeder ET, et al. Effects of pharmacological doses of nandrolone decanoate and progressive resistance training in immunodeficient persons infected with human immunodeficiency virus. J Clin Endocrinol Metab 1999 Apr;84(4):1268-76.
82. Hassager C, Jensen LT, Podenphant J, et al. Collagen synthesis in post-menopausal women during therapy with anabolic steroids or female sex hormones. Metabolism 1990 Nov;39(11):1167-9.


SPINAL FLUID
83. Damkier HH, Brown PD, Praetorius J. Cerebrospinal fluid secretion by the choroid plexus. Physiol Rev 2013;93(4):1847-92.
84. Kiiski H, Aanismaa R, Tenhunen J, et al. Healthy human CSF promotes glial differentiation of hESC-derived neural cells while retaining spontaneous activity in existing neuronal networks. Biology Open 2013;2(6):605-612.
85. Whendon JM, Glassey D. Cerebrospinal fluid stasis and its clinical significance. Altern Ther Health Med 2009;15(3):54-60.
86. Weller RO, Djuanda E, Yow H, et al. Lymphatic drainage of the brain and the pathophysiology of neurological disease. Acta Neuropathol 2009; 117:1-14.
87. Csarr HF, Harling-Berg CJ, Knopf PM. Drainage of brain extracellular fluid into blood and deep cervical lymph and its immunological significance. Brain Path 1992; 2:259-296.
88. Laman JD, Weller RO. Drainage of cells and soluble antigen from the CNS to regional lymph nodes. J Neuroimmune Pharmacol 2013; 8:840-856.

89. Rydovik B, Holm S, Brown MD, et al. Diffusion from the cerebrospinal fluid as a nutritional pathway for spinal nerve roots. Acta Physiol Scand 1990; 138:247-248.

GENETIC COLLAGEN DISORDERS
90. Henderson FC, Austin C, Benzel E, et al. Neurological and spinal manifestations of the Ehlers-Danlos Syndromes. Amer J Men Gen 2017;175C:195-211.
91. Castori M, Voermann NC. Neurological manifestations of "Ehlers-Danlos Syndromes. Iran J of Neurol 2014; 13:190-208.
92. Sevesto S, Merli P, Ruggier M, et al. Ehlers-Danlos Syndrome and neurological features: a review. Childs Neuro Syst 2011; 27:365-371.
93. Schievink WI, Gordon OK, Tourje J, et al. Connective tissue disorders with spontaneous spinal cerebrospinal fluid leaks and intracranial hypotension: a prospective study. Neurosurgery 2004;54(1):65-71.

AUTOIMMUNITY
94. Wang L, Wang FS, Gershwin ME. Human autoimmune disease: a comprehensive update. J Intern Med 2015; 278:369-395.
95. Zweiman B, Levinson AI. Immunologic aspects of neurological and neuromuscular diseases. JAMA 1992;268(20):2918-2922.
96. Meisel C, Schwab JM, Prass K, et al., Dirnage U. Central nervous system injury-induced immune deficiency syndrome. Nat Rev Neurosci 2005;6(10):775-786.
97. Javidi E, Magnus T. Autoimmunity after ischemic stroke and brain injury. Fron in Immunol 2019; 10:1-12.
98. Tennant F. The physiologic effects of pain on the endocrine system. Pain Ther. 2013 Dec;2(2):75-86.

RISKS
99. Epstein NE. The risks of epidural and transforminal steroid injections in the spine: commentary and a comprehensive review of the literature. Surg Neurol 2013;4(supe2):574-593.
100.Eisenberg E, Goldman R, Shclag-Eisenberg D, et al. Adhesive arachnoiditis following lumbar epidural steroid injections: a report of two cases and review of literature. J Pain Research 2019; 12:513-518.
101.Nelson DA. Dangers from methylprednisolone acetate therapy by intraspinal injection. Arch Neurol 1988;45(7):804-806.
102.Kitson MC, Kostopanagiotau G, Alimeric K, et al. Histopathological alterations after single epidural injection of rapivacaine, methylprednisolone acetate, or contrast material in swine. Cardiovasc Interven Radiol 2011;34(6):1288-1295.

Made in the USA
Lexington, KY
03 November 2019